PRAISE FOR
THE 100-YEAR GOLFER

"I don't know anyone who embodies the spirit of the game of golf like Ilchi Lee. He understands that the game is one of potential . . . the potential to create the next great shot, to learn from each shot, and to find the joy of being in nature in pursuit of that little white ball. He plays with total joy, and I believe it when he says he will play till he is 100!"

—**Dave Bisbee,** Director of Golf, Seven Canyons Golf Club,
United States

"This book reminds us that training the body and mind is a shortcut to better golf. It presents practical meditations and unique exercises that are helpful to golfers of any level, along with the inspiration to make golf part of a deeply fulfilling life. *The 100-Year Golfer* is a gem that gives good mental stimulation to golfers regardless of age or background."

—**Sangho Choi,** South Korean golfing legend,
Holds the record for most wins in KPGA history

"These days, it's common to obsess over the mechanics of the swing, but Ilchi Lee's book approaches golf through breathing and energy. It was so refreshing to read, like discovering a clear spring on a hot day. I hope that many golfers read it and come to understand the greater depth and potential of golf."

—**Heon Kim,** Principal of Happy Golf Training Center,
South Korea

D0913627

"This book struck me like I had been hit with a bamboo stick. I was thinking of dropping golf as I'm approaching 70. After reading this book, I added "playing golf in good health until the age of 100" to my bucket list. This is a remarkable guide that inspires golfers who want to enjoy the benefits of increased longevity and continuous challenge. If this book is followed, you will be able to shoot your age."

—**Sooin Kim,** Golf columnist and the author of
Power Golf, South Korea

"I was pleasantly surprised at Ilchi Lee's enlightening insight into golf and its potential to help us grow and learn more about ourselves by being in the present moment. As I approach the beginning of a new season, I am inspired by the idea that I'm gaining a deeper connection with myself and that a sport that I love can help me grow as a human being, rather than merely pursuing the next win."

—**Nicola Madden,** Hilton Park Golf Club Ladies Club
Champion, Scotland

"As I watch the devastating effects of dementia on my mother, I have never valued mental and physical health more. Reading Ilchi Lee's *The 100-Year Golfer* offered a blueprint on how to keep your mind active and your body in shape to enjoy the game well into old age. Who wouldn't want that?"

—**Matt Callcott-Stevens,** Writer for *GolfSpan* and
Golf Workout Program, South Africa

THE

100-YEAR
GOLFER

THE
100-YEAR
GOLFER

7 Arts for a Lifetime
with the Game

ILCHI LEE

BEST
LIFE
MEDIA

BEST
LIFE
M E D I A

459 N. Gilbert Rd, A-275
Gilbert, AZ 85234
www.BestLifeMedia.com
480-926-2480

First paperback edition: June 2022
Library of Congress Control Number: 2022933433
ISBN-13: 978-1-947502-22-2

Cover photo © iStockphoto.com/vm

To a mind that is still, the whole universe surrenders.

— Lao Tzu

Table of Contents

SECOND ART: FITNESS
Fitness Is Golf Power

THIRD ART: BREATHING
Develop Your Golf Mentality with Breathing

FOURTH ART: MEDITATION
Get into the Zone with Relaxed Concentration

FIFTH ART: QIGONG
Create Your Own Swing with Qigong

SIXTH ART: SELF-HEALING
Bring Self-Care and Self-Healing to Your Golf

SEVENTH ART: CONSCIOUSNESS
Consciousness Determines the Quality of Your Golf Experience

PART 3
Golf and Life

Golf for a Better Life, a Better World

Only a decade ago, many people would have laughed at me, incredulous, if I'd said that I plan to play golf until I am 100 years old. But now that more and more people are living past 100, walking the fairway at that age is no longer a pipe dream. Of course, this is not an easy goal, but that is what makes it worthwhile.

Five years ago, I published the book *I've Decided to Live 120 Years*. The book isn't just about having a greater lifespan but also about leading a healthier, happier, more fulfilling life and achieving the life goals we've chosen. It's about making longevity a blessing to those around us, and to the world, as well as to ourselves.

It's an established fact that people today on average live much longer than our ancestors did. The question is not so much if but how we will live those extended lives. This golfing book emerged out of my desire to find ways to turn this intention into action, and through my experimenting with and exploring the possibilities of a 120-year life.

When I was young and looking for my purpose in life, I tested the limits of my body, and I searched my consciousness for what it was I really wanted. I devoted myself to taekwondo, hapkido, and other martial arts beginning in adolescence, hoping to deal with the confusion and emptiness that came from my unanswered questions about life. In my late 20s, I began serious spiritual practices, feeling that I couldn't go on without an answer to the question of who I was. In the end, I found my answer. And through that answer, I discovered the immense spirit and creative power of the human brain and body.

After finding my answers, I created a mind-body training program called *Dahnhak*, known as Body & Brain Yoga in the United States. This practice consists of methods based on the ancient Korean tradition of *Sundo*, and it is meant to help people who—like me—want to know the purpose and meaning of life and who want to develop the infinite possibilities of the human brain and body.

Later, I integrated brain-related knowledge and information into my program, creating the Brain Education system. Realizing that many institutions study the brain biologically and medically, but few research how to apply their findings in daily life, I established the Korea Institute of Brain Science and two universities. The goal was to develop a practical application of knowledge about the brain into an academic discipline.

I believe that the brain is the key to developing individual potential and creating a sustainable, peaceful world. As a result, I have committed myself to developing and sharing methods that allow people to increase their quality of life through better use of the brain.

Why I Love Golf

I first picked up a golf club in my early 30s, and I've been playing for almost 40 years now. Like many golfers in South Korea, I started playing to meet people and to make connections. Later, though, I fell in love with golf, coming to enjoy the game itself.

One of the reasons I enjoyed golf was that it truly challenged me. When I first started, it didn't go nearly as well as I'd thought it would. Golf hasn't given me generous scores just because I'm an expert in qigong, meditation, and brain training, someone who has been studying the human body and consciousness for decades! I'll be honest up front: I'm no golf prodigy. Even after 40 years, I'm still a bogey player.

Shooting 100 when I expected to break 90 left me feeling humbled. Experiences like that pushed me beyond curiosity, giving me the attitude of a researcher, a seeker. Golf made me reflect upon myself, challenging me to stay committed to my goals. It trained me, enabling me to think flexibly and creatively amid unpredictable change. I came to love golf even more because the concentration, composure, and confidence required for this mental sport, the conscience and consideration emphasized by the gentlemanly spirit of the game, the respect for companions and nature, and the required constant training of body and mind are all consistent with the values pursued by Brain Education.

Since golf has fascinated me, I've long thought of writing a book combining this game with the mind-body training of Brain Education. Twenty-five years ago, I created specific exercises for golfers to help develop the senses required for an effective golf swing. Inspired by a dream, I even designed a putter. Now, in my 70s, I'm finally publishing a book I've been thinking about since my late 40s. Only now, it seems, is my golf allowing me to write this book.

I am neither a professional golfer nor an expert golf instructor. I'm merely an amateur golfer who loves the game. I taught myself to play golf and experienced a lot of trial and error, thanks to my own stubbornness, which kept me from listening to what others had to say. Golf has given me opportunities to develop patience, self-control, and self-discipline—either as a punishment for my obstinacy or as a reward for my persistence. I'm grateful for that and find it comforting.

To beginners, however, I wouldn't recommend learning golf on their own. I'd tell them to learn the basics well by taking lessons from a good pro. But I would recommend to anyone that they enjoy golfing freely in a way that's right for them, without being tied down by the forms or specific styles of others. Once you reach a certain level, golf inevitably becomes a self-taught sport, whether or not you had a mentor at first. It's your responsibility to control your body and develop and master your senses; you have to study and train yourself.

About This Book

The 100-Year Golfer isn't a systematic introduction to golf or a manual of techniques. There are plenty of those available in print and online. Rather, this is a book for sharing tips that have helped me improve my game and ideas I've gained through my personal golf experience and the Brain Education techniques I've long studied and taught. Instead of writing about golfing skills, I've included methods for training body and mind and enhancing the connection between them for a lifetime of enjoyable golf. In writing this book, I kept in mind serious golfers who consider the sport a tool for lifelong self-discipline, not merely a sport or hobby.

This book is divided into three parts.

Part 1 addresses a mental attitude for enjoying golf for a lifetime. If you're a golfer, whether in your 20s, 40s, or in your 70s like me, imagine yourself golfing in good health throughout your life—and while you're at it, picture yourself golfing at 100. You can lead a more fulfilling life if you look at the whole of your life and design it with a long-term perspective. The same goes for golf. If you make up your mind to golf in good health until you're 100 years old, taking care of your body and mind will be essential. You'll end up thinking about the meaning of golf in your life, and you'll develop your own philosophy for the game.

Time is a precious asset in our finite lives. Golf is a game that requires more time than other sports, so if you plan on playing golf your whole life, you might as well make that time a little more valuable. Try making golf a spiritual practice for training your body, brain, and spirit, and a lifelong study of the mind. In Part 1, I've included my thoughts on how to make golf truly enjoyable by playing golf that is naturally suitable for you, and how to spend a lifetime growing through golf, communing with yourself, your companions, and nature.

In Part 2, I've introduced Ilchi Brain Golf, a method of training body, mind, and spirit for golfing to 100. I've covered principles and practices from Brain Education that golfers will find helpful, dividing them into seven arts: energy, fitness, breathing, meditation, qigong, self-healing, and consciousness. Of these, the most basic is *qi*, energy. From Korea's ancient Sundo culture, I have applied the secrets of sensing and moving qi to help create the ideal physical and mental state for golfers. You'll learn how the core energy principles of Brain Education can improve your golf, and you'll discover practical tips and advice immediately applicable to your game. I've also included stories of golfers who have applied principles of Brain Education and various mind-body training methods to their golf.

In Part 3, I've shared some life wisdom that golf has taught me, along with memorable golf experiences and meaningful thoughts I have about the golf game I've been dreaming of. Think of them as stories told by a friend as we walk the fairway together.

Golf and our lives aren't separate. We bring to the course things we've learned in life, and we bring to life things we've learned on the course. One of the things I've realized through golf is that a good golfer is also a good person. Golfers who do their best to be their best every moment, rather than trying to be better than others, have a noble air about them. They are the kind of golfers who respect and care for their companions. These character traits reach beyond the golf course, pervading their work and daily lives.

I've traveled the globe teaching Brain Education, meeting countless people from different backgrounds and cultures. In the process, I've become convinced that, deep in their hearts, all human beings have a passionate interest in and love for life and for the world. We are at our greatest when we work for the sake of others and for a better world, rather than merely for ourselves. Within us are hearts that understand the value of all lives, hearts longing to create a more peaceful, sustainable world.

I believe that such desires and longing may be expressed and nurtured through golf, and that golf helps make better people and a better world. If you golf regularly, you've enjoyed such benefits from society and nature, and you can influence those around you. Whatever your situation, I hope that golf can help you use your power in a more fulfilling and beautiful way.

Proposing Brain Sports

Many of the concepts and techniques introduced in this book are relevant for various fields beyond the golf course. If you're doing sports in addition to golf, I suggest that you use the contents of this book for those pursuits as well. You can apply the seven arts of Ilchi Brain Golf to all activities that use your body and brain, including swimming, running, basketball, archery, tennis, baseball, etc. This is why I've proposed the concept of "brain sports," and I'm continuing to research and experiment, applying the principles and methods of Brain Education to more sports.

Brain Sports is focused on developing the true potential of the human brain through sports. This doesn't just mean improving your skills and abilities in order to win more games. Brain Sports is an effort to expand the value of sports beyond competitive measures, where only a few elite individuals can hope to challenge the limits of human physical potential. Instead, I would like to see a world where everyone is encouraged to reach their full holistic potential, to seek the balance of mind and body, and to develop courage, confidence, empathy, and creativity through sports.

This book is an attempt to express my ideal of Brain Sports through golf. Because it is a lifelong sport that can be enjoyed by people of all ages, not only by energetic young people, golf is perfectly suited to the purpose of Brain Sports. I hope you will enjoy golf as a Brain Sport that fosters and illuminates the great spirit and character in the human brain.

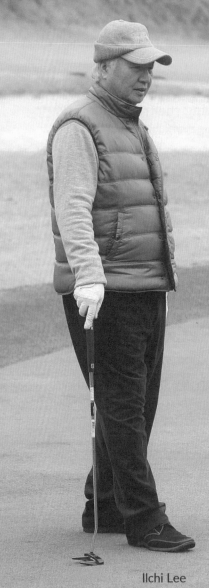
Ilchi Lee

PART 1

Dreaming of Becoming a 100-Year-Old Golfer

Jongjin Lee

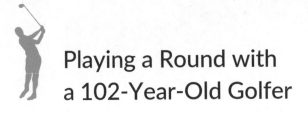

Playing a Round with a 102-Year-Old Golfer

One chilly winter morning, I planned to meet with a very special person to play golf. The temperature was a little below 40°F, but on the golf course—located on a vast, empty plain—it felt even lower, like it was around freezing. The 102-year-old Jongjin Lee showed up with his son wearing simple, comfortable clothing, joining another golfing friend of mine and me on the teeing ground. There were also video and photo crews who would record our round of golf.

After warming up, Jongjin stood on the tee box. Everyone watched his first shot, gasping in surprise. It was the first time any of us had ever seen someone older than 100 in person, so we couldn't help but be excited to witness him coming onto the course and taking his first swing.

I wondered what he felt as he saw all of us standing there, holding our breath, eyes focused on him. Setting up his shot, Jongjin looked back at our party and said, "You've all come out to watch me, I see." His joke and our laughter released the tension.

He adopted a stable setup posture, paused for just a moment, and hit his drive. Everyone in our party cheered—"Good shot!"—and applauded. He sent the ball flying 140 yards. That distance would've been short for a young golfer, but his swing, with such a stable posture, was miraculous for someone at the age of 102.

After everyone hit their tee shots, we were about to pile into the golf carts, following the caddy's instructions. But Jongjin waved us off, saying he would walk. We were all shocked. The frost hadn't yet melted, making the grass rather slippery. I was worried; Jongjin would be in big trouble if he slipped and fell. The whole party suggested that he take a golf cart, but he refused. "I'm happiest when I'm walking on the golf course," he said, taking the lead down the fairway. "Why come here if I'm going to ride in a golf cart?" Embarrassed and left with no other choice, everyone followed him.

Jongjin's 66-year-old son, who was golfing with us, said he has weak knees and sometimes takes a golf cart when he goes out on the course with his father, who walks 18 holes with ease. While playing a round, I even felt short of breath a few times on a somewhat steep uphill slope. Amazingly, Jongjin showed no signs of struggling. The round of golf, which was initially supposed to go only nine holes in consideration of Jongjin's age, went all 18 holes.

I carefully watched his swing and every move he made throughout the round. Jongjin's drives ranged from about 140 to 165 yards. He made great approach shots and putts, carefully examining the terrain around the holes and the slope of the greens. On most greens, he never needed more than two putts. His body was neither strong nor flexible compared to those of us in our 50s and 60s who played the round with him, but there was something inexpressible in his swing. Despite the limitations of a body worn out over a century, his swing was smooth, balanced, and beautiful. It suddenly occurred to me, "Oh, he's doing the most perfect swing he can right now!"

Another thing that left a deep impression on me was the relaxed attitude Jongjin showed throughout the game. He lightened and brightened the mood with his wit and gentle humor. When I took off my hat for a commemorative photo with Jongjin, he saw that my hair was whiter than his. "Oh, wow," he said. "I should call you 'big brother.'" Facing each other, we burst out laughing.

Jongjin Lee regularly shoots his age. During a commemorative golf outing for his 101st birthday, he shot 89. Earlier in his life, he was a successful businessman and athlete. At one point, he even won 10 consecutive national soft tennis championships in South Korea. Jongjin started playing golf relatively late, at the age of 54, and instantly fell in love with the game. He became a single handicap player within six months of beginning golf, thanks to his tremendous concentration and practice. In his prime, his skills gave him a handicap of eight.

After our round, this is how Jongjin answered my question about how his game went:

"In the past, getting a birdie was easy. Now, though, it takes four or five strokes to get the ball on the green. I stopped worrying about the number of my strokes a long time ago. Now I'm happy walking the course on my own two feet, enjoying a good time with the people playing a round with me, like today."

The round of golf with Jongjin Lee that day had been arranged at my request. I had come across an article about him in a South Korean newspaper while collecting resources for a book on golf at the time. His story—the 101-year-old "age shooter"—immediately caught my attention. Setting a date and thinking of playing a round of golf with him excited me, making my heart pound like I was a little kid looking forward to summer vacation.

There was another, more personal reason I planned to play golf with Jongjin. At the time, my father was 89 years old. Once healthy and active, he had started declining rapidly in his mid-80s. He seldom went out of the house and spoke so little that at times he didn't say a word all day. "Dad, I want to see you live long and in good health," I would say every time I saw him. "I've lived long enough," he would reply. "I get no more pleasure in living; it's now time for me to go."

It was sad to see Dad like that, just waiting helplessly for the day he would die, having lost all will to live. After meeting the golfing centenarian, I wanted to show Dad photographs of Jongjin playing golf and share his advice on health in old age. I wanted to give my father new hope and motivation.

Looking back now, I see that I was the one motivated by the encounter with Jongjin, not my father. Watching him bring joy to those around him, walking and golfing 18 holes while past the age of 100, made me think, "Golfing long and in good health is also an art."

I've Decided to Golf until I'm 100

I was 62 when I met Jongjin Lee, and I had been playing golf for almost 30 years. The game had become an important part of my life; I enjoyed my golfing skills, which were growing day by day. Though my age was increasing, my strokes were decreasing, and my immersion in the game was deeper than ever before. I hadn't always golfed a good game, but I felt pride and joy in learning something new about myself and about golf with every round I played.

Common sense suggests that golf would be more physically demanding now than when I was young, but that hasn't been true at all. By the time I walk to the ninth hole, my legs hurt a little and my lower back and shoulders ache a bit, but by the time I finish 18 holes, my whole body feels relaxed and full of energy—as if it had never ached at all. When golfing alone, after finishing a round, I sometimes even play another nine or 18 holes.

I had thought that I wanted to golf for a long time even before I met Jongjin. Until then, though, it was just a vague notion. You occasionally see a golfer in her 80s but rarely in her 90s; I had thought that people could golf to 90 only if they were especially blessed.

After meeting Jongjin, though, and with all the talk about so many more people living past 100—the stuff you read in the newspaper or see on TV—it really hit home for me. Golfing with someone older than 100 opened my eyes to the possibilities. It made me realize that the tale of the centenarian golfer, once only a dream, could emerge among my friends, and that I could even be the protagonist in that story.

Just thinking about such possibilities gave me a sense of exhilaration and joy. I realized once again how deep my affection for golf was. I really love golf! Besides work and people, golf is the thing to which I've most consistently devoted myself. My ambition surged; if I can golf as long as I want, I'd like to make my game a more meaningful, more valuable experience.

I made the conscious choice to play golf to the age of 100 in order to turn those possibilities into my own reality. I also came to dream of shooting my age—playing a 100-stroke game at the age of 100. As I mentioned in the introduction to this book, I've also chosen to live 120 years. I set the **maximum number of years scientists claimed was possible for humans at the time as my intended lifespan. I did this as a way of redefining old age for myself. From this perspective, the 'second half' of my life is a time when I can complete the** dreams I've chosen.

At first, the thought of living to the age of 120 and golfing to 100 was incredibly strange. Neither of these ideas was the result of scientific calculation. They were just my choice, my resolution, and I'm well aware that it won't be easy. But the more I studied and reflected on both the potential lifespan and the golf lifespan of humans, the more confident I became in thinking that it wasn't impossible and could become a reality for many people.

I've found new research to support my thinking. A study published in May 2021 in *Nature Communications* indicates that humans could live up to 150 years. It seems like the numbers increase once every few years. Big tech companies are even looking for ways to cure death with a vision of creating near-immortality. I think we can't and shouldn't try to remove death from our lives, but I firmly believe that we can live a healthy, fulfilling long life. And our choices play a big role in that picture.

Choosing to play golf to the age of 100 wasn't only an expression of my will to stay healthy and fit enough to play the game my whole life. It was a personal promise to explore myself and life through golf, which has gained greater meaning for me the closer I've examined the sport. It is also a pledge never to give up my hope for tomorrow and my absolute positivity toward my life and golf.

For many long-time golfers like me, the game is more than a hobby or a way to stay healthy. Golf is an exciting game that makes me feel happy, a form of meditation that helps me look deep into my mind. Golf not only signals the condition of my body and mind, but it sometimes also acts as a healer offering me a remedy. It's a teacher awakening me to the wisdom of life, a friend with whom I share my solitude— something I can share with no one else.

I've been studying and training my body for all my life, but since setting my golf-at-100 goal, I've been devoting myself more seriously and wholeheartedly than ever before to training my body and brain. In addition to qigong, meditation, and breathing—already a part of my life—I've increased my strength training. I try to develop my muscle strength and endurance whether I'm working, sitting in an office, or driving in a car, moving my body whenever I get the chance. Now that I think of golf as a study and practice that will be with me my whole life, I'm more grateful for it, and it feels more precious. Heaven willing, I'm hoping my body will continue to cheer me on as I work to achieve the dream I've chosen: becoming a 100-year-old golfer.

Make It Your Goal to Play Golf Your Whole Life

Jongjin Lee is not the only example who can inspire us to be golfers at 100 and beyond.

America's oldest PGA member, Gus Andreone, used to play nine holes three times a week until a few months before his death at the age of 107. He had eight holes-in-one in his lifetime, the last when he was 104.

On the European KLM Open Tour celebrating its 100th anniversary in 2019, a 100-year-old German woman, Susan Hosang, played with the pros on the 13th hole. The image of her hopping onto the tee box, making her shot, and then smiling brightly was broadcast on television worldwide. One golfer said he was shocked at how quickly Susan walked up to the green when he played with her that day. She had been 70 when she began playing golf.

Golf legends Jack Nicklaus and Gary Player are now in their mid-80s. They've retired as professional players, but they still hit the first tee shot every year at the Masters and are active as golf businessmen. Remember the nude photos Gary Player showed in ESPN magazine when he was 77? The pictures revealed that, at the time, he had the slim physique and solid muscles of a 45-year-old. He still plays every day at the age of 86.

Most golfers have a goal for their number of strokes. If you haven't been golfing for long, you'll probably want to break 100. Depending on your own golf experience, age, and physical condition, you might have different goals, like breaking 90 or 80, becoming a single-digit handicapper, a scratch player, or shooting your age. But have you ever thought about your golfing lifespan? How long do you want to golf, until what age—70, 80, 90, 100 years? I'd like to suggest that you add one more goal to your golfing objectives: playing golf for the rest of your life.

In the past, longevity was a gift bestowed on only a few; now it has become a blessing enjoyed by many. So why can't we play golf to 100 and beyond? Choosing your golf lifespan is far removed from the kind of arrogance that would go against nature or the will of God. Just as we set goals for growth and development in various areas of life and do our best to achieve them, we need to have a proactive attitude toward our golf lifespan.

Instead of saying, "It would be good if I could golf until then" or "I'll try," you might as well make up your mind: "I will golf until that age." It would be even better to establish a concrete goal, like playing a round at some golf course to celebrate your 90th birthday. If your kids and grandkids also play golf, it would be especially meaningful to set the goal of having three generations play a round together.

There is a subtle but fundamental difference between "I'll do it" and "I'll give it a try." When you say you'll give it a try, you can't use 100 percent of your energy, because your mind doesn't come together entirely behind your goal. Your brain knows that there's uncertainty in your mind. Conversely, deciding resolutely to do something will give you more confidence and take a load off your mind. You *can* use 100 percent of your energy, because there's no confusion or conflict within you. If you make up your mind to do it, your brain will get everything ready, making all the preparations necessary to achieve your goal. Amazingly, your environment will also start changing, conditions developing in a direction that supports your choice.

Of course, choosing our golf lifespan doesn't fully guarantee that we'll stay healthy and be able to golf until that age. But if you proactively manage your body and mind, using your free will and passion—the greatest gifts given to humanity—the probability increases that you'll be able to golf long and in good health.

Compared to other sports, golf isn't too much of a burden in old age. As we get older, though, our shot distance decreases and our stroke number increases, leading many to think about setting aside their golf clubs. But that doesn't have to be the case. Jongjin shot 89 at age 101, and Canadian golfer Arthur Thompson shot his age at 103, setting the world record for the oldest player to shoot his age. I often hear stories of people who celebrate their 100th birthday by playing a round of golf with their friends and family. Many of the golfers I've met didn't start playing golf until they were in their 60s. With some people picking up golf for the first time in their 70s or 80s, why would you need to give it up just because you're getting older?

Your Choice Really Matters

I recently met another older person, one who had turned 100 a few months back. A Korean member at the Body & Brain Yoga center in Auckland, New Zealand, had come to know a centenarian at the local Korean American Association and contacted me to say there was someone I should meet. I was in Kerikeri, New Zealand, at the time and was glad to meet this individual, so I went straight to Auckland.

Inmyeong Kim showed up wearing orange pants and a cool denim jacket. It turned out that he was a passionate practitioner of Body & Brain who had started training in the late 1980s, in the early days when I was teaching it in South Korea. He told me he had been practicing daily, continuing to take good care of his health after immigrating to New Zealand with his family more than two decades ago. Even now, at the age of 100, he reads without reading glasses and, amazingly, still drives a car!

I looked at Inmyeong's physical condition. As if to say "This is a piece of cake," he sat down, spread his legs wide apart, bent forward at the waist, and grabbed onto the ends of his feet. His half-lotus and other postures—like clasping his hands behind his back or lying on his back and bringing his knees to his chest—were better than those of most 50-somethings. Although he doesn't golf, he has the strength and flexibility to do a good-enough swing. He's a welcome model of longevity, confirming that we can live active, healthy lives regardless of our age, depending on how we take care of ourselves.

Believe that you can play golf in good health for a long time. No, better yet, choose to do it! What's important here is resolve. That means making up your mind, resolving to do something. All success begins with a choice. Not everything works out automatically just because you make up your mind to do something, but *nothing* happens unless you do. Deciding to become something or do something, setting a goal, and ceaselessly challenging yourself, striving to achieve that goal—this is the great character and power of the human brain.

"If you choose it, it will happen." This is one of the principles I believe to be most important for using the brain. When we truly choose something, our brains work to achieve it. If a method for achieving what we've chosen doesn't exist in the world, our brains will sometimes invent one for themselves. Sooner or later you'll get close to your chosen goal if you focus and work hard without giving up.

Next time you stand on the golf course, seriously ask yourself some questions. How long do I want to play golf, until what age? Observe how this question and your answers change your golf game with an open mind.

Bring Joy to Your Golf Intentionally

What kind of golf can you play your whole life? What mindset do you need to golf until you're 100 years old? Thinking about the characteristics of golf at 100, I've organized them into three categories: joyful golf, natural golf, and connecting golf. This is the kind of golf I want to continue playing as long as I have the strength to lift a club, as long as nature allows.

More than anything else, golfing to the age of 100 should be joyful. A lifelong sport should be one you enjoy. Many people, especially in South Korea, start golfing to entertain business partners, to make connections, or to socialize with friends. Though they may begin with such motivations, the reason they end up as long-term golfers is probably that they have fun playing. "Amateur" means lover of something, someone who engages in a pursuit because he enjoys it, not someone who does it as their primary occupation.

Still, even those who golf because it's fun feel a lot of stress while playing. Unlike those of other sports, golf skills aren't easy to maintain at a certain level. No matter how hard you practice, it's normal for your play to seesaw wildly, depending on your condition, the weather, your companions, and your mental control that day.

This also goes for famous professional golfers. Golf king Tiger Woods set a personal worst for an official tournament, hitting 10 strokes on a par-3 hole in the final round of the 2020 Masters. The ball went in the water twice in a row, the next shot flew over the green and into a bunker, and the shot from the bunker went over the green and into the water again. In the world of golf, even professionals who've lived on the golf course for 10 or 20 years can suddenly fall into a slump one day.

When you first get into golf and start feeling the thrill of a well-placed shot, you'll be so excited that you'll wonder, "Why didn't I know it was so fun before now?" You'll soon learn, though, that golf doesn't always go as you'd like. Balls that go right where you want them on the practice range will hook and slice on the course, or your friends' skills improve nicely while you seem stuck in a rut. The stress feels severe at times like these, making you want to drop golf altogether and causing you to ask yourself, "Why did I ever start this?" But one well-placed drive or successful long putt will send a thrill through your body, instantly blowing away such regrets and leading to a tug of war between love and hate for the game.

Rare is the golfer who has never experienced this tug of war. The game feels like a heavy burden when it gets bad, rather than being enjoyable. You become obsessed with the fantastic swings or distances achieved by the pros, or you compare yourself with others, working yourself up over your scores. At such times, golf becomes a stress machine instead of an energizer. But to enjoy golf your whole life, you need to make a conscious effort to put your health and happiness first. If you're injured, irritable, angry, or continuously anxious because of golf, you can't make a lifelong game of it.

One day I was playing golf early in the morning in Sedona, Arizona. Sedona is a desert, so they water the grass on the golf course a lot, sometimes making the ground too wet and the ball difficult to hit. On this day, the ground felt especially sloppy. My tee shot was good on the first hole, which was a par 5, with the ball landing in the middle of the fairway, but it took four iron shots to get it on the green. I duffed the ball, the head of the iron going into the wet ground, and on top of that, the wind was against me, keeping the ball from going in the desired direction. I felt my chest tightening, my breathing becoming irregular.

It was evident that I wouldn't be able to play a good game in that state. So I controlled my breathing, inhaling deeply into my lower abdomen. And I asked myself, "What attitude are you going to have for your next shot?" I decided to maintain a good mood regardless of the results, considering every ball precious, being grateful and devoted with each shot. I made up my mind to have fun regardless of whether my shots went where I tried to put them.

Thinking that way, I was able to maintain a stable, comfortable breathing rhythm throughout the game. My swing felt smooth and relaxed. That day I played one under par. With my skill level at the time, I usually played 10 to 12 over par.

You probably have your own routine before starting a round, like stretching to warm up or controlling your breathing. In my experience, the most crucial thing in a pre-round routine is adjusting your mental attitude, deciding how you'll approach the game. Of course, having a joyful attitude doesn't mean you'll always get a good score. Sometimes, I end a game with a bogey on all holes, and other times a double bogey. You'll definitely improve your game, though, regardless of your score, if you make up your mind to maintain a positive attitude no matter what.

It's essential to decide what kind of golf you want to play that day before standing on the first tee and then to remind yourself of that frequently during the game. It will be easier to move past any mistakes if you make up your mind to play an enjoyable, happy game of golf. That's not likely, though, if you approach the game thinking, "I need to beat my partner no matter what."

It's not easy for anyone to play this game to their satisfaction. But being upset and annoyed every time things don't go your way isn't good for you or your partners. Even when the ball doesn't land where it should, you need to create good feelings and be grateful that golf keeps you on your toes, always striving to do better. Emotions naturally arise based on your environment, but you can also create them for yourself. While you automatically smile when you feel good, you'll feel better if you deliberately smile and laugh even when something bad happens.

A golfer who—along with Tiger Woods—has an 18-hole record of 59 strokes and a season average of 68, Annika Sörenstam said the following in an interview on a South Korean golf TV channel:

"My distance has decreased a little since I retired. It's only natural that someone who doesn't practice a lot isn't going to golf as well as someone who does. Lower your expectations for yourself and have fun playing. I mean, that's what I'm doing. Have fun like me."

Having fun means you can be okay even when you make mistakes. You play your game, recognizing, "Ah, this is where I'm at now." We need to remember that golf is a *job* for pros but a *game* for us amateurs. To enjoy golf as a form of play, you should respect golf and be kind to the game. If I get mad at the ball, my clubs, the golf course, etc., golf will get mad at me. If I get on golf's bad side, I am not going to do well, no matter how much I want to succeed. So, when I miss a shot, I just think of it as the game not being ready to reward me because I haven't respected it quite enough! Then, I consider what I did to hurt its feelings and try to improve. Approaching my game in this way makes golfing fun and light, never too serious.

Your Golf Is Not You, but Yours

A long time ago, I taught Brain Education to a young professional golfer in South Korea. At the time, she was in such a bad slump that she couldn't participate in any tournaments, and she came to see me after being introduced by her high school coach. When I asked what golf meant to her, she replied, "Golf is everything to me." So I gave her some advice.

"If golf is everything to you, then you're bound to become controlled by it. Golf should be a means for creating happiness and direction in your life; you'll end up living in a hell of stress if golf itself becomes your life. When your golf game stops going well, you instantly feel empty. Whether or not you're golfing well, you can sustain your game only if you feel your own confidence and freedom."

If you want to enjoy golf your whole life, you should prioritize the health, happiness, and inner satisfaction you get from the game, not golf itself. Didn't you start playing to be healthier and happier, not golfing for golf's sake? "I realized that golf shouldn't be my whole life," confessed beloved South Korean golf empress Se-ri Pak herself after emerging from a prolonged slump.

Once you decide to experience golf as a happy, enjoyable game, you can laugh at and encourage yourself when you're feeling impatient because your skills aren't improving as much as you'd want, and when you're disappointed that you don't achieve the distance you used to. You can enjoy golf when you're playing well and when you're not. You can also end a round after only nine holes, not needing to go 18. If you can't get out on the course, you can just practice at a golf range. You can enjoy golf according to your particular environment and situation.

The words most often heard by beginners in Brain Education are "My body is not me, but mine," and "My mind is not me, but mine." This means that I should use my body and mind, own them, not be led about by them.

You can apply the same idea to golf. "My golf is not me, but mine." If you identify with your golf game, you'll degrade and diminish yourself when you hit one out of bounds or duff a shot. One swing at a time, golf jerks you around—making you feel good one moment, only to make you suffer the next.

The 100-Year Golfer

But if you think "My golf is not me, but mine," you take a step back from your game, gaining perspective, and you're able to use golf to increase your quality of life.

Golf itself doesn't make us happy or unhappy. Instead, the game brings us happiness or unhappiness depending on how we deal with it. I think golfing with humility and gratitude, and, more than anything else, with a joyful heart, could be the secret to playing long and well.

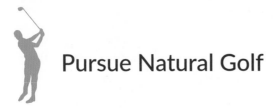

Pursue Natural Golf

Each of us golfs under different conditions. Age, physical condition, psychological state, pattern of adapting to circumstances, and living environment are different for all of us. Golf swings are said to be like fingerprints, different for each golfer. So you should golf in a way that's natural to you, without trying to imitate somebody else.

Famous for having a unique swing, Inbee Park, who has been the number one ranked player in the Women's World Golf Rankings on four separate occasions, once said in an interview, "I do a light backswing without being bound by a complicated swing mechanism. Being fast doesn't make a swing rhythm good. It's important to swing naturally with your own rhythm."

Park said that although she's learned a lot about the swing from famous coaches known worldwide, being bound by an overly mechanical swing seemed to make her lose her natural rhythm. So she studied her own body, developing a swing that was right for her, with her low flexibility and weak wrists compared to other players.

She probably doesn't mean that it's okay to swing a club any which way just because you're playing your own game of golf. She means that you should thoroughly learn the basics of a good swing and observe and study your own body, finding a natural swing that's right for you instead of imitating the best golfers. There are numerous techniques for perfecting golf swings. What's important is that no matter how good the technique, you need to find one that's right and doable for you.

Two of the people I've played rounds with have deeply impressed me. One was the 102-year-old golfer Jongjin Lee, mentioned previously, and the other was a famous South Korean comedian, Gookjin Kim. When the pandemic restricted my activities at home in New Zealand, I happened to watch Gookjin's golf channel on YouTube. Fascinated by his swing, I wanted to play a round with him. Our schedules worked out when I was visiting South Korea to lecture in 2021, so we set a date to play golf together.

Gookjin has a unique swing, utterly different from the form commonly taught by coaches. He looks relaxed and casual when he hits the ball, without tension, but his shots are accurate and fly far. While we rounded all 18 holes, I sensed solid internal energy in him as he consistently swung without shaking. He hit the ball comfortably and naturally. His swing didn't feel forced at all. I wondered how much he must have practiced to get that level of naturalness into his body. He probably did a great deal of research, going through repeated trial and error, to find an effective swing that was right for his physique. I was happy and grateful to encounter a good model of natural golf in the pleasant rounds I played with the humble, considerate Gookjin.

Gookjin's swing is natural and suits him. It certainly wouldn't look natural for me if I were to imitate it. I have a natural rhythm that's all my own. The task of golfers is to find the swing that's most natural and suited to *them*.

Being natural also means golfing within your personal strength and ability limits. If you get greedy, trying to go beyond that, your golf will be unnatural. Looking at the swings of pros who send the ball flying more than 300 yards, you'll see that, while they're very powerful, they don't seem to take a lot of force and look effortless. However, they've practiced millions of times to get those swings. Behind the seemingly casual strokes of a skilled calligrapher and the light footwork of a seasoned dancer are hundreds of thousands of hours of sweat-soaked effort.

Without considering your physical condition or ability, try imitating the great, full swings of the pros—with their excellent rotational power and big arcs—and you'll just end up ruining your body. It's hard to make good use of high-difficulty techniques unless they're supported by elite strength and flexibility.

Suppose you usually do three pull-ups. You can do up to three naturally. Put your mind and muscle into it, and you might be able to knock out four or five with fairly good form. From the sixth repetition, though, grimacing and writhing, you'll attempt the exercise using a form others find hard to watch. The same goes for golf. Getting greedy beyond your natural level of strength and skill will ruin your swing, sending the ball flying off to all the wrong places.

There is the naturalness of the body in its 20s and the naturalness of the body in its 70s. Past 60, you can maintain your muscle strength through regular exercise, but your agility declines. Reacting swiftly to stimuli or quickly changing the position or direction of your body doesn't feel as easy as it once did. To play natural golf, you have to respect the environment of your changed body and adjust your movements and approach to the game accordingly.

Let go of your desire to play the same game of golf you played in your 30s with your 60-year-old body. Of course, every once in a while you might have such a round. You can't golf that way all the time, though. A senior golfer will hurt herself if she tries to keep golfing the way she did when she was young, without considering her changed physical condition and flexibility, or if she gets greedy for distance. The disappointment might break her heart even more, perhaps even making her want to give up golf. What's worse, if she feels frustrated by being older, she'll feel discouraged and frustrated in life as well as in golf.

Golf is a living thing. It accurately reveals the condition of your body whenever and wherever you play. Accept your condition as revealed by golf and play in a way that's right for you. I'm not saying you should always be satisfied with the status quo and never hope for more. What I *am* emphasizing is that although you should establish a goal and tenaciously challenge yourself to achieve it, you cannot play golf beyond the skills and abilities you've developed through practice.

I want the golf I play to resemble nature. Unadorned nature radiates beauty at every moment. The rising sun is amazing, but the setting sun is also beautiful. Flowers in full bloom on a sunny spring day excite the heart, but winter trees, their bare branches exposed, send echoes reverberating deep in the heart. An oak tree doesn't try to become a pine tree. It just strives to grow as a beautiful oak tree.

Just as the flowers, trees, and birds of the forest have different colors, sounds, and feelings, each of us has our own rhythm and energy. We feel joy when we're free to express our own colors, feelings, and inspirations. That uniqueness inside us is expressed through our golf swings. When you swing your club in the way that's perfect for *you*, you feel at one with your swing, which manifests naturally and without awkwardness. You have your own balance and harmony because your naturalness is expressed, even if your swing lacks the form of a pro. And so those watching also feel beauty in it.

If I play golf like nature, whatever my age or condition, no matter whom I play with or on what course, in every moment I can play my game in the way that's right for me. Though my physical skills decline with age, I can continue perfecting my natural golf using both the experience I've accumulated and a more mature attitude.

How scary is it when a baby first learns to walk, staggering and tottering around? As she grows, though, she gradually develops her own natural gait. We can recognize friends from far off by the way they walk toward us. Each of us also has a golf swing with a unique style and rhythm, much like our gait. Natural golf is the game you can play best in your present physical condition, with *your* skeleton, muscle strength, and flexibility. No one else can teach you naturalness. You have to find, feel, and create it yourself, for it is a rhythm unique to you—one you can share with no one else.

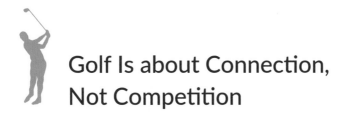

Golf Is about Connection, Not Competition

With golf, I want a game that continues to grow even as I get older. What is growing golf? If the number of your golf strokes decrease, is that growing golf? It's impossible to play a game that grows throughout your lifetime if you think your score is all that matters.

It's true that golf is one game in which you can improve your skills even in old age, reportedly making it the only sport in which a 60-something can beat a 30-something. Even my own golf skills are much better now than when I was in my 40s.

But sooner or later, the distance of your driver shot will decrease, and it'll take you four or five shots to get the ball on the green. If you play competitive golf, which is obsessed with scores and winning, your passion for the game will cool as the number of your strokes increases. The more you play, the more it will feel like you're going downhill, and you're unlikely to want to keep playing for long.

I believe that connection is the key to lifelong growth in golf. You can grow with your game throughout your life by connecting with yourself, your golf partners, and nature on the golf course. Golf becomes more enjoyable when you focus on connection, not your number of strokes.

The most important object of connection in golf is yourself. Is there a better sport than golf for connecting with yourself? Golf is an honest game. Of course, all sports call for honest sportsmanship, but there are no referees in golf. The golfer is his or her own referee.

Each and every shot immediately reveals the state of the golfer's body and mind. You can see yourself through the naked honesty of golf. It's not just posture or body habits of setup, swing, approach, and putting. Golf shows us our hearts. It shows us being impatient or hasty, and it shows us losing consideration for others because of our desire to win. Unforgiving of even a single millimeter of error, the pitilessness of golf is stressful, but its mercilessness—involving neither interest nor emotion—is like a mirror reflecting back to us an image of who we are.

At times the golf ball feels like God to me. God is pitiless— pitiless but not heartless. Were nature bound by small affections, it would disrupt the cycle of life. The leaves of spring and summer must fall without regret before winter comes if new leaves and flowers are to bloom the next year. The pitilessness of nature is thus a great love and blessing. The pitilessness of golf teaches us humility and keeps us examining ourselves and striving to be better.

In golf, another person's play does not directly affect mine, as it does in soccer or basketball. This game lacks the concepts of offense and defense against an opponent. Nobody intentionally drops your ball in a bunker or water hazard. You play your game with your ball. Even if you have an opponent, it's essentially a solo exercise. Still, the psychological impact that your partner's play has on your game is formidable. The nature of the game is such that it makes us look more deeply within ourselves. We've all probably had the experience of unwittingly losing our usual swing rhythm when a partner hits a long tee shot, and we stagger as we try to hit the ball farther than the other guy.

Golf is a highly introspective game. That the sport has this character, however, doesn't mean that everyone gets to know themselves better by playing golf. To see, you must *try* to see, and to understand better, you must try to learn.

Golf becomes a great mentor if your attitude pushes you to study and train your body and mind while connecting with yourself through the game. You will be able to better observe the habits of your mind—the way you respond emotionally, your attitude toward others, how you deal with crises. The better you know yourself, the more your powers of self-regulation grow. In golf, self-regulation is a skill.

If we can connect with and develop ourselves through golf, the game will always bring us the joy of growth, whether we are 20 or 100. Our bodies change along with our ages, but that always brings us new things to learn and know, suitable for our changed physical environment. In middle age, I practiced to increase my distance; now, though, I'm searching for the kind of golf I can play in a way that's most natural for my 70-something body. At 100, I think I'll be working to develop the simplest, least strenuous swing.

One of the joys of golf is playing together. At first you start with close friends or acquaintances; later, though, you have more opportunities to play with people you're meeting for the first time. When you golf together for four or five hours, the character—both strengths and weaknesses—and unadorned personality of each person are laid bare. Some people inspire admiration with their manners and etiquette; others disappoint with their self-centeredness and pettiness, turning out not to be who they'd seemed to be.

Just as all shots, both good and bad, can teach us and make us grow, everyone we meet on the golf course can be our teacher. Some are considerate of others, positive in everything, a joy to play with. Some throw a fit every time they miss a shot, upsetting the people next to them. Some use obvious tricks, making you never want to golf with them again. All are mirrors reflecting me—for they could all *be* me.

If you wish to be a gentleman or lady on the golf course, you should be strict with yourself and generous with others. If you always do the opposite, no matter how long you've played golf or how well you score, instead of being a gentleman, you'll just be stubborn and self-centered.

Once when I went to play golf with my family, my wife teased me. "You're usually so impatient," she said, "but coming to the golf course turns you into Confucius." Golf draws out the qualities already in us, both good and bad, amplifying them. If I'm going to play golf my whole life, it would be great if I could say and hear others say that golf has made me a better man.

In my South Korean upbringing, I learned about the five virtues humans should have: benevolence, righteousness, courtesy, wisdom, and sincerity. Benevolence is compassion, empathizing with the pain of others. Righteousness is ashamed of injustice and seeks to protect what's right. Courtesy is respectful and considerate of others and is humble. Wisdom knows how to differentiate between right and wrong. And sincerity encourages trust by turning words into deeds acting on what is said.

Golf is a great sport for developing the five virtues, and for meeting and learning from people with different backgrounds, personalities, and experiences. As much as you grow by struggling with your golf game, so, too, you learn and grow by meeting, influencing, and being influenced by people on the golf course.

Golf without Winners and Losers

Is noncompetitive golf possible? It's easier said than done. It is challenging to play golf without the thought of winning. Pro golfers engage in blood-curdling competition, immersing themselves in levels of stress difficult for the rest of us to imagine. That's the life they've chosen. Amateurs don't need to do that, though. Wouldn't it be great for me to play my game and my partner to play his, cheering each other on as we do?

I want to play golf for completion rather than competition. Instead of focusing on winning, I dream of a kind of golf in which players endlessly challenge themselves, striving to perfect their game. In competition, there are winners and losers, but in completion, we find the satisfaction and joy of everyone striving to be their best. Even if we called together all the immortal golf heroes we love, none would say that their golf has reached completion. They merely keep learning, studying, and striving to improve a little at their own level of golf experience and skill.

Thus, I don't like betting on golf. If I bet, my desire to win interferes with my composure and makes it difficult to sincerely cheer on others. I might occasionally make a bet with close friends, with the loser paying for a meal. But if you want to play as a form of self-cultivation, it's best to distance yourself from betting, which encourages the development of a gambler's mindset. Moreover, there's no reason to bring to the golf course a worldly culture that motivates us to deceive ourselves and others, and to occasionally use sabotaging strategies in order to win.

It may be difficult for energetic young golfers to imagine golf or any other sport without winners and losers. If you're a senior golfer in the latter half of your life, though, you can dream of the kind of golf that lets you relax your once-clenched fists, even letting go of your desire to win. If you decide to keep golfing after the age of 60, then your game becomes a relationship with yourself, not a competition between yourself and others.

Some readers may ask what fun golf is without winners and losers and without betting. But you can find pleasures in golf other than the fun of winning: the joys of beating your score from the last round, of developing and improving your golf; the joys of growing together and sharing frank discussions about life, inspired by the good shots and manners of companions; and the joys of learning in nature, which changes with the seasons and shows the undaunted power and beauty of life even amid impermanence.

"Golf will grow as long as it's fun," said Tom Watson, who achieved 39 PGA Tour victories and shot his age for the tenth time at the age of 70. Those who find it fun and rewarding to commune with themselves, their companions, and nature, who consider golf a form of self-discipline, will keep golfing and growing even when they reach the age of 100.

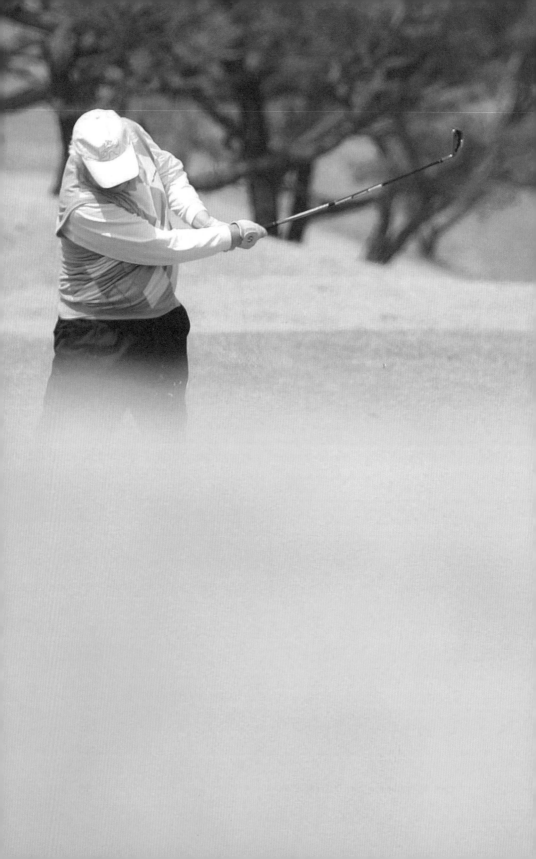

PART 2

Seven Arts for a Lifetime of Golf

Why Seven Arts?

I'd like to propose seven arts that anyone can learn and develop for a lifetime of golf that's joyful, natural, and energetically connected. These seven arts are energy, fitness, breathing, meditation, qigong, healing, and consciousness. I call them "arts" because I believe these practical skills add new beauty and meaning to golf. I've organized the content of this book based on Brain Education principles and programs, so I'm calling it "Ilchi Brain Golf."

If you think of Ilchi Brain Golf as a house, then energy and consciousness are its cornerstones. Energy and consciousness are the keys to improving any activity you perceive and experience through your brain, which of course includes golf. Fitness, breathing, meditation, healing, and qigong can then be called the five pillars of Ilchi Brain Golf. As you develop these seven arts, you'll find yourself unlocking new awareness and abilities on the golf course. Best of all, you'll discover new ways of practicing, playing, and improving your game while also upgrading your overall health and wellness.

These seven arts are well known beyond the game of golf, but you may be surprised to discover how much they can empower your golf experience. For example, we all know that being fit can help your golf game, but did you ever think that golf can help you get a better sense of how to be fit? And, while we all have experienced moments of beautiful harmony with nature on the golf course, have you embarked on your own meditation practice in order to find this feeling more often? When you use the seven arts to improve your golf game, you'll no doubt see benefits in your daily life as well.

If you want to upgrade your game, I want to encourage you to consider the role of your brain. You do more than think, analyze, judge, and focus with your brain. Physical activity is essentially controlled by the brain, so whatever you do with your body, you're doing with your brain. To play well, your physical condition, technique, and psychology need to support your game. Every golfer who's played at least a few rounds knows the negative impact that mental stress, lack of focus, and frustration can have on physical performance. Even your practice habits, muscle memory, and ability to learn new techniques are ultimately determined by your brain. Thus, you can view them as an extension of your mind.

While many of us strive to develop physical and psychological skills for golf, there's another piece of the puzzle: the bridge between the physical and the psychological, between the mind and the body. There's an aspect of your being that connects tangible and intangible skills, enabling them to support each other. It's energy and consciousness, the cornerstones of Ilchi Brain Golf.

For the past 40 years, I've been teaching methods for developing and using the potential of the human brain through Brain Education. One of the stereotypes I've encountered most frequently is the idea that brainpower equals intellectual ability. This capacity, however, is but a fraction of the brain's infinite potential.

People often focus on the intellectual ability of the brain when deciding who's "smart," but I believe that harmony and creativity are actually the most important and are key to creating a happy, successful life. These two brain abilities complement each other like yin and yang. Creativity is like the masculine principle of yang, allowing us to make positive changes in our lives and in the world. Harmony, on the other hand, is like the feminine principle of yin, allowing us to cultivate an internal state of emotional and mental equanimity. Together, these abilities allow us to return to a state of emotional and physical balance, despite external forces that constantly threaten to derail us, while also giving us the ability to find new solutions to life's challenges and opportunities.

Isn't this the essence of golf? No matter how much we understand golf intellectually, our swing won't improve unless we can creatively implement new mind-body operations and harmonize them with the fundamental swing we've already created. Nurturing a sense of harmony and creativity is the core of Brain Education. To improve your golf skills and have joy, be natural, and feel connected when playing golf up to age 100, you need to develop these two brain abilities.

The sense of harmony can also be called a sense of balance, a sense of equilibrium. This includes emotional, mental, and spiritual harmony and equilibrium as well as the simple physical balance of the body. The brain knows when body and mind are out of balance and has a natural tendency and ability to restore equilibrium. That's why our pulse, blood pressure, body temperature, and other vitals are kept constant even though we don't think about them, and why our bodies exhibit the natural power to heal themselves when they are injured or ill. Though our lives are surrounded by constant change, we can maintain continuity, stability, and order because of this sense of harmony and balance. Golf, perhaps more than any other sport, tests this equilibrium with every shot. By developing your power to find harmony and balance, you'll optimize your golfing potential no matter the situation.

Equanimity, the ability to maintain a sense of harmony and balance is an innate ability that every human brain has as a part of its nature. When your sense of harmony is restored, you can find inner peace and stability even though your external environment is challenging. This sense isn't relative, coming and going under the influence of external conditions. It is an absolute sense within you that never disappears and cannot be destroyed under any circumstance. You can achieve the physical balance, mental composure, and natural swing that's essential for good golf when your sense of harmony is awake and maintained. The seven arts of Ilchi Brain Golf will help you develop a sense of harmony in a way that you probably haven't experienced before.

After harmony, the second most important brain capacity is creativity. The greatest weapon in his golf, Tiger Woods has said, is the creative mind. Every golf game presents unique situations, even if you always play on the same course. One day you may find the course soft and inviting, with barely a hint of a breeze at your back and the rough cut down nice and low. The next week you could be teeing off into a 20-mph headwind, the fairway rock-hard or dotted with puddles, the rough mercilessly gobbling up errant shots. The spot where the ball lands changes with each swing. You must make the best choices you can at every moment, considering the terrain and wind as well as the distance to the hole.

Our brains have intuition, insight, and wisdom greater than the knowledge, experience, and information we've accumulated over the years. Such intuition and insight develop in people who trust and challenge their brains instead of setting limits for themselves. If you rely solely on knowledge or experience, you become addicted to learning. Some think they can't do anything without learning it from someone else, feeling anxious or even guilty unless they do just as they've been taught. Certainly, you can learn from an expert to improve your golf skills. What's more important, though, is to go beyond formal learning, to keep exploring your own body and mind, striving to find and refine your own swing. You must connect what you know in your mind with what you do with your body. This is the essence of Ilchi Brain Golf.

Will and passion are the keys to awakening creativity in the brain. Many people have fantasies about creativity, thinking that it is when an idea suddenly flashes into the brain one day. But the biographies of creative people are not stories of "suddenly one day." The "aha!" moment of inspiration comes in the instant of brain integration when the knowledge and experience you've accumulated interconnect with your brain's intuition and insight. Ceaseless planning, challenges, and trial and error lead to the moment when the light suddenly switches on in the brain. Creation doesn't happen without concentration and immersion in what you're doing, or without will, passion, and strong execution.

Your will and passion to achieve your chosen golf goals are the fuel enabling you to draw maximum power and resources from your brain with every shot. Many people, especially at the practice range, end up hitting shot after shot with limited focus or intention. Then when they get onto the course, their minds are ill-prepared for the novel circumstances in which they find themselves. To play golf well, you need to have a creative mind. What makes creative golf possible is an attitude of never giving up—of taking up the challenge and somehow finding a way, even when you encounter a bad lie, bad bounces, or get stuck in a spot with seemingly no way out.

Rather than golf techniques, Ilchi Brain Golf teaches methods for training your body and mind and strengthening the connection between the two so that you can play your best golf in good health for a lifetime. I've tried to include practical tips and advice for helping you develop your brain's sense of harmony and creativity. I want to help beginners fully experience the joy of golf by optimizing their ability to learn and adapt, and to help seasoned golfers by increasing their sense of energy and self-awareness. Through golf, we can understand our bodies and minds more deeply and get one step closer to unraveling the mysteries of life.

Each of these arts can help you create a new taste, style, and rhythm in golf and in life. I hope the advice and stories you'll find in the following pages will help you transform your golf into an art of the highest order, using your brain's harmony and creativity.

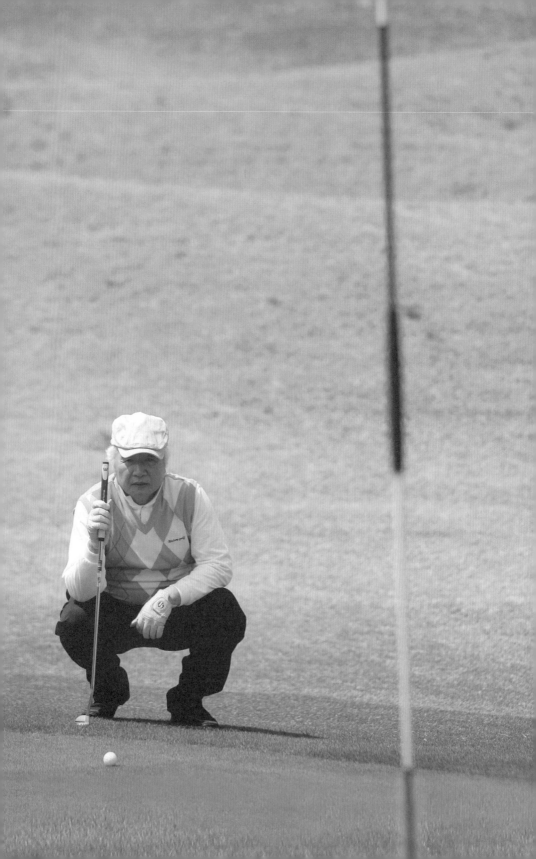

Sense Energy
to Make Golf
More Fun

From Thinking Golf to Feeling Golf

G olf is played with the senses—by feeling, not thinking. When you're playing well—even if you don't think much about your swing—your backswing, downswing, impact, and follow-through all happen naturally as a single motion, smooth as flowing water. Worrying about each component of the swing just adds tension to your movement, likely resulting in a missed shot.

"Feel the rhythm and tempo of the swing." "Feel the weight of the clubhead." If you're a golfer, you've probably heard these expressions countless times. Most golfers, though, find it tough to feel their body and feel their swing while playing the game. If you've spent hours on the practice range honing your swing, only to be shocked at the awkwardness when you watch a video of yourself, you're not alone. It's incredibly difficult to apply what we know and see to the way we move, especially for something as complicated and subtle as a golf swing.

To make things even more difficult, we all develop habits. The longer you play, the more those habits become ingrained.

Even though you try to change your motion and implement a new swing technique, old habits inevitably reassert themselves. And finally, physical injuries and limitations can restrict our ability to change. Your body simply may not be able to copy certain movements.

All these things—a lack of awareness, past habits, and physical limitations—can prevent you from improving your golf swing. When you think about it, these same factors affect our lives as a whole, limiting our ability to adapt and grow. If you've found yourself repeating the same mistakes over and over despite knowing that you've made them before, you're probably suffering from one or all of these three factors.

Set aside feeling your body for a moment. What about feeling or observing your mind while you play golf? Are you aware of your thoughts, emotions, and actions during a round, and can you control them before negative thoughts or emotional impulses ruin your play? Or do you throw your club in rage after missing a shot, taking your anger out on your blameless caddy, only to regret it later? For most golfers, having a clear awareness of the mind's activities probably seems more challenging than feeling the body.

Self-awareness—carefully observing and feeling your own actions, thoughts, and emotions—is a critical ability for improving the quality of your performance in all areas of life, including golf. Once you are fully self-aware of your swing and bodily movements when golfing, you'll naturally go on to the self-correction stage. For example, if you notice that your arms and shoulders are stiff and you don't feel the clubhead because your grip is too tight, you'll try to correct it. But you can't even think about solving your problems if you don't really notice them in the first place. Unfortunately, many golfers lack self-awareness, so their game doesn't improve, and they repeat the same mistakes again and again. That was true for me, too, when I was a novice golfer.

Rather than simply watching more YouTube videos, spending hours grinding on the practice range, or buying expensive lessons (all of which can be helpful but won't solve these problems), I want to introduce a new idea: work on your mind-body connection.

We always *seem* to be there with our bodies and our minds, but often this isn't really true. Our bodies have nowhere else they can be but here and now. Our minds, though, move around, going from place to place as they follow nearby sensory stimuli, information, thoughts, and emotions instead of being at one with our bodies. Sometimes they go into the past, sometimes into the future. But you won't have a good feel for your golf swing unless your mind is focused on your body. Strengthening the connection between your body and mind means calling your wandering mind back into your body, here and now, keeping your mind and body in one place.

Develop Your
Energy Sense

Most golfers focus on a certain swing thought, which is supposed to help them move their body correctly when they swing. But often they can't really feel their body, meaning it's difficult to discern where the tension is or where the motion is interrupted. How can you better feel your body and mind when playing golf? How can you better connect your body and mind? As the answer, I want to suggest using your sense of energy. Mastering and training your sense of energy can help you develop more feelings in your body, which naturally leads to a better swing.

When I refer to energy (also called *qi*, *chi*, *ki*), I'm talking about the energy of life. It's what connects consciousness and the body. It's the phenomenon that lets us know we're alive. And through various practices, we can make it strong and healthy.

You've probably already experienced what I'm referring to. If you've ever found yourself in a mental and physical state where relaxed concentration, physical power, and emotional contentment seem to coexist in balance, you're familiar with the optimal energetic state.

By developing your energy sense, you can get a better feel for the subtleties of your body posture, muscle movement, and coordination in each part of your swing, address, and putt. In addition, by controlling your energy, you can relax your mind while playing and focus on the goal you want. When you're nervous or anxious, maintaining the feeling of energy for just two to three minutes will calm your mind, balance your brain waves, and make your breathing easier.

I'm willing to say that 90 percent of improving your golf game comes from strengthening your mind-body connection rather than from studying new techniques or tricks. That's right—your own mind and body are the keys to getting better at golf. Veteran golfers will benefit even more than beginners from strengthening the mind-body connection because they've already accumulated plenty of mechanical know-how from books, videos, instructors, and watching professional golf on TV. Of course, beginners with a stronger mind-body connection will be able to progress more easily and accurately from the start. You develop a subtler, richer feel for golf when you add a sense of energy, strengthening the connection between your body and your mind.

Using your energy sense, you can improve the effectiveness of your practice. How your mind and body are functioning will make or break the habits you create through those hours of practice. If your training is impacted by a lack of awareness, obstructive habits, or physical ailments, you won't improve as much as you could. But swinging as if you were doing qigong or tai chi—feeling the flow of energy inside and outside your body—will let you focus better on your practice. And, because you are in touch with your body's condition, you can minutely adjust your movements and avoid most injuries caused by overexertion.

Using your energy sense to play golf not only connects body and mind, but also lets you feel and commune with your brain more deeply. Since the mind is an operation of the brain, you are essentially training your brain when you learn to sense and control your mental state. There's no way to move or feel your brain as you do your hands and feet, because your brain has no muscles or sensory nerves. The most direct means for feeling and interacting with your brain are the senses of energy and imagination. Through energy, you can be aware of and feel even those areas that are out of reach of the five senses.

Develop Your Touch in Golf Using Energy

For most people, the hands are the most sensitive part of the body. By sensitive, I don't mean ticklish. I mean that most people have more sensation and awareness in their hands than in any other part of their body. So, it's natural to practice sensing with your hands. In golf, too, the sensitivity or "feel" of the hands is critical.

Players with a good "feel" or sensitivity have a valuable advantage over those who just mechanically go through the motions. Golf instructor and former pro player Butch Harmon once said that what set Tiger Woods apart from his peers was the incredible sensitivity he has in his hands.

Can sensitivity be developed? I think so. Try the following energy sensing exercise.

Begin in a comfortable sitting or standing position. Straighten your spine and relax your shoulders. Rub or clap your hands for 30 seconds to get the blood flowing. Then tap your fingertips together for 10 seconds. Next, shake your wrists for 10 seconds. Rub your hands one more time. Now you're ready.

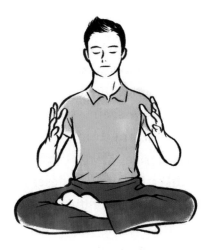

Hold your hands out in front of you, palms facing each other with about 3 inches of space between them. Keep your elbows slightly away from your rib cage to avoid dulling the sensitivity of your hands. Breathe comfortably and focus on your hands. What sensations do you notice? Is there warmth or tingling? Pulsation or pressure? Do you feel a magnetic sensation between your hands?

Now gradually and repeatedly move your hands closer together and then farther apart, concentrating on the sensations between them. Does it feel like a weak, tingling electric current or like something heavier, such as magnets in the palms of your hands pushing and pulling on each other? Does it feel lumpy like soft cotton candy or as if your hands are moving slowly, immersed in water? If so, your "sense" is waking up. Practice this, and you'll be able to maintain a magnetic sensation as you move your hands more freely. The feeling may expand through your wrists and arms, all the way to the core of your body. Do these movements for about three to four minutes, and then lower your hands onto your knees.

When you watch an advanced martial artist or tai chi practitioner, you may notice the fluidity and balance of their movements. What you're seeing is their deep mind-body connection and the strength and flexibility cultivated through years of practice. Martial arts introduce energy sensing practices like the one I've described above, which can help anyone develop this ability.

As you practice this energy-sensing exercise, you may realize that feeling energy supports a lot of well-known putting tips. For example, having "soft hands" makes a lot of sense when you want to maintain a feeling of energy during the putting stroke. Relaxing your arms, letting them hang from your shoulders, also helps you maintain an awareness of connection with your hands. Finally, maintaining a connection between your arms and body helps you sustain the feeling of energy and minimize excessive arm movement in the putting stroke. Simply put, the more you can feel your hands, the more you'll be able to sense and control what the putter is doing.

Golf with a Cool Head and a Warm Belly

Which should be cool and which should be warm, your head or your abdomen? Intuition and experience teach us that our heads should be cool and our bellies warm. Stress flips this balance, heating your head and cooling your belly. This puts you in a daze, keeping you from thinking clearly and preventing your organs from operating smoothly, making you feel stuffy and bloated. Only a cool head and a warm belly create an energy balance that allows all the body's organs to function well. In traditional Korean medicine, this energy balance is called "Water Up, Fire Down." This principle tells us to keep our heads cool and our bellies warm by letting the energy of water rise and the energy of fire sink.

Water Up, Fire Down is the ideal energy state, allowing our bodies and brains to function at their best. Consequently, it creates the best mental and physical conditions for playing golf. With your head cool and your belly warm, you can come up with the best golf strategies and make stable shots.

To cultivate Water Up, Fire Down, you need to build the energy center in your lower belly, developing sufficient power there. In fitness training, this energy center is commonly called the "core" or "power zone." Physically, it's the body's center of gravity; energetically, it's the seat of the most fundamental life force in our bodies. When your energy center is strong, your head cools and your belly warms. Your body from your belly button upward is "emptied" of energy, which gathers instead in your lower body and produces the condition called "empty upper body, full lower body" in traditional Korean martial arts.

A fundamental principle of energy training and martial arts systems such as yoga, qigong, and tai chi, "empty upper body, full lower body" applies to the game of golf as well. When adopting a setup posture, you should relax your upper body, shoulders, arms, and grip and find your balance in your lower body, lower back, legs, and the soles of your feet. Only if you create a sturdy, stable posture—balanced in your lower body and the energy center in your belly—can you move your spine freely and your upper body flexibly to make a solid swing.

"In your address, point your belt buckle at the ball on the tee." "When finishing, point your belt buckle at your target." Both of these standard tips are saying to focus your attention and load your center of gravity into your energy center.

If you usually do exercises for feeling and strengthening the energy center in your belly, when you address the ball, your lower body will feel like a tree putting down deep, strong roots. Your lower body should be solidly planted on the ground, and your upper body should be empty. Only then can you achieve a powerful swing, your upper body pliable like willow branches bending in the wind.

These days—for various reasons—many of us suffer from a reversed energy flow, making our bellies cold and our heads hot. I don't need to tell you that this won't be great for the quality of your game. But if you haven't experienced the power and clarity of Water Up, Fire Down energy circulation, you might not realize what you're missing. Golfing with a hot head and a weak belly is a shortcut to slices, hooks, and high scores. If your energy rises to your head instead of staying in your belly and lower body, you'll be tense before your shots, your head clouded by distracting thoughts. In that condition, you won't be able to feel your core during your swing, and you'll lose strength and balance, shaking and swinging without consistency. Such a state also consumes a lot of energy, which will wear you out and sap your concentration even after nine holes, making you sloppy for the rest of the round.

Are you able to keep your awareness grounded in your core and maintain calm even after missing a short putt or duffing an approach shot 20 yards from the green? Or does the heat rush to your head, making your face red with embarrassment or anger, and causing your legs to lose their strength? Keeping a cool head on the course can save you multiple shots every round.

The ability to sense energy and Water Up, Fire Down are closely related. While you can use exercise, meditation, and breathing to develop Water Up, Fire Down circulation even when you can't feel energy, your power to maintain Water Up, Fire Down grows if you develop your energy sense. You can quickly recognize the signs of disruption in your body's energy balance and take necessary action to restore Water Up, Fire Down circulation. With a water hazard in front of you, you can immediately notice when your hands holding the iron are sweating and your heart is pounding, and you can use three or four deep breaths to sink the energy into your lower abdomen and calm your mind.

All the exercises and training methods introduced in this book will move your body into a state of Water Up, Fire Down based on energy principles. In particular, the Intestinal Exercise (introduced in the following fitness chapter), Brain Wave Vibration (meditation chapter), and abdominal breathing (breathing chapter) are surprisingly powerful if practiced consistently. These exercises will contribute to your health and longevity as well as to your golf game.

Self-Coaching: Me Watching Myself

To help you understand how greatly energy can sensitize the body and mind, I want to talk about how I first came to feel energy and what changes I experienced as a result.

In my late 20s, I went to an old bookstore in Seoul in search of a book to study. It was a place I often frequented to find books on martial arts, ancient philosophies, and oriental medicine. Looking through the bookshelves, I noticed a volume with half its cover missing and found myself picking it up. It was about tai chi. When I flipped through to the middle of the book, these words caught my eye: "Mastering energy makes you invincible."

Hit by surprise in that instant, I took a step back. An intense tingling instantly shot through me like an electric shock. My whole body trembled. "Eh, what is this?" Without a moment to think about what was happening, as my trembling subsided I felt something warm and comfortable enveloping my whole body like a fog. My mind calmed down, and I felt reverence without understanding why. The peace was incomprehensible.

Quietly closing the book and putting it back in its place, I left the bookstore and headed for home. I moved cautiously as I walked and got on the bus, fearful that even a tiny distraction would make the feeling disappear. When it was time to sleep, I got into bed quietly; I wanted to get up the next day with that same feeling. I fell asleep thinking that I should get up and meditate at 4 am.

When my eyes opened the following day, I checked the time. It was exactly four o'clock, not a minute off. I got up—actually, it's more accurate to say that my body got itself up—and headed toward a mountain behind our neighborhood. It wasn't *me* going; my *body* was going. It felt like some unseen power was moving me. The instant I'd thought I should look at the book, my hand had stretched out to where it was. The same happened when I ate. My hand wasn't lifting the spoon; it seemed like some power was raising my hand. Such movements felt very natural. My body wasn't tense anywhere, and at times all my motions seemed very slow, as if I was watching a slow-motion video.

I later realized that the powerful force I experienced then—the true nature of what was wordlessly moving my body—was energy. Although I had known about energy through hapkido, taekwondo, and many books I'd read, that was the first time I had powerfully experienced it with my own body.

One of the significant changes that happened to me after I experienced energy was that I sensed another self watching me. This felt vivid and clear, like watching a movie about what I was thinking, what emotional state I was in, what actions I was performing. And I was changing myself, not just watching. The self watching me encouraged my ordinary self, sometimes scolding and sometimes coaching, leading me to make better choices.

The energy sense can have a similar effect on your golf. In short, your awareness of your body and mind in golf grows, making self-coaching possible. Once you start applying the energy sense to your golf, you can maximize the effectiveness of every practice and every game you play.

There are many things to say about energy, but here is one that I want you to take to heart: ultimately, your energy condition is due solely to your choices, your actions, and your attention. Of course, we face challenges from other people, from our environments, from life's situations, but in the long run, it's our own choices, actions, and attention that create our energy condition. The "me watching me" that I experienced—that is, my consciousness—is the entity regulating my energy. Energy and consciousness form an inseparable whole, which is why they are the cornerstones of Ilchi Brain Golf.

TESTIMONIAL

Relax and Develop Control through Energy Training

By Baegyeong Seong
67-year-old man, Jeju Island, South Korea, 20-plus years of experience

I worked for a long time on Jeju Island. There were a lot of golf courses nearby. The broad grass fields of the golf course, the oxygen, sunlight, and walking... all helped me manage my health. What's most important in golf is consciously controlling your body. Doing energy training for 20 years, I was able to develop a sense of that relatively easily.

Before swinging, I would command my body, "Fix your lower body, relax your upper body, and keep your head fixed." These are the basics known to all golfers, but following these principles is not always easy—you end up hitting a top ball if your lower body rises even a little or you stare at the ball. Having given such commands, I'd feel the energy going down to my fingertips.

Feeling energy means relaxing. You'll get distance on the ball only if you relax. Your body will tense up the moment you think with your head, trying to get a good stroke. You can send the ball as far as you want only if you swing while feeling your body, focusing only on your body.

You keep getting distracted unless you feel your body. When you're golfing, if the guy next to you tries to distract you, saying, "Oh, there's a hazard ahead," your awareness goes to the hazard even though you try not to think about it. But if you feel the energy at times like that, you'll focus on your body, and your awareness will come into your body. And you can golf comfortably and consistently, not easily shaken even by somebody trying to sabotage your game.

After energy training and meditation early every morning, I do putting practice and swing-visualization training. I practice for a short time, about five minutes, but it's very effective when my body is relaxed and my brain waves are stable, so I'm sticking with it. When I'm on the course moving for my next shot, walking, I choose what number club to use and how big to make my backswing; then I bring up an imaginary screen in my brain, where I picture myself swinging. I also do regular strength training, including walking 10,000 steps and doing squats and calf raises.

Even though I can't get out on the course often, thanks to energy training that I've learned from Ilchi Lee's Brain Education, I'm easily able to maintain my low-80s handicap. "My body is not me, but mine." Constantly training to apply this basic principle to my golf has been a big help.

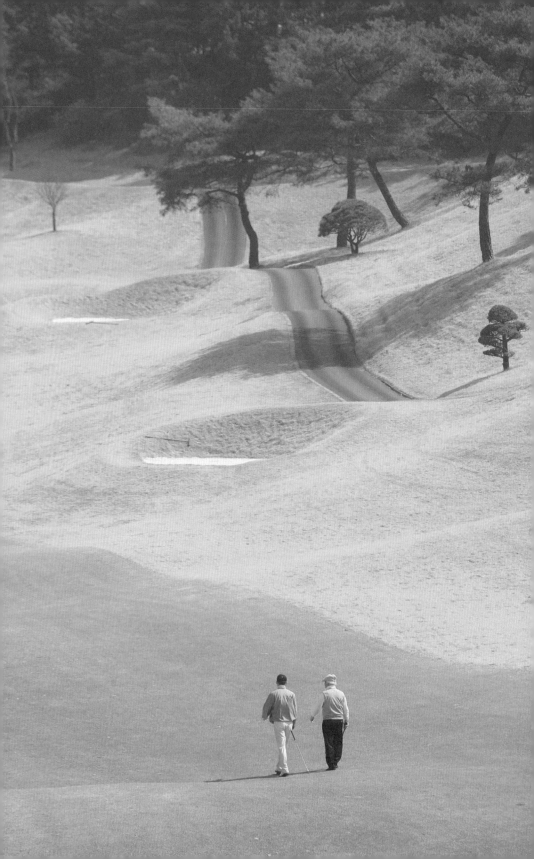

Fitness Is
Golf Power

Your Body Is Your Most Important Golf Equipment

The famous South African pro golfer Gary Player, age 86, is nicknamed "Mr. Fitness." As mentioned earlier, many were shocked when a nude photo was released of a muscular Player, taken at 78. Many people suffering from a chronic lack of exercise and addiction to fast food are said to have started exercising because of him. Even now, he stretches every day and trains his muscles from head to toe. In particular, he does a thousand sit-ups a day to avoid losing his core strength.

Player achieved a Grand Slam—winning all four majors— not only on the PGA Tour but, after turning 50, he also did so on the Senior Tour. He gives his exercise-honed body as the reason for his success, stressing that you should exercise no matter what if you want to enjoy golf when you're older.

"You have to keep moving. If you're just sitting around watching TV like an old man in the back room, you're doomed. If it's hard to make the time, invest just two minutes a day in the morning and evening. If they only do 100 sit-ups before they get up and 100 before they go to sleep, an average amateur golfer will have a much better core for their age, and they'll score much better than they do now."

I can't help but agree with Gary Player. Your most important piece of equipment in golf is your body. You can replace other equipment if it wears out or doesn't fit your hand, but you can't do that with your body, right? If you want to play golf your entire life, you need to put incomparably more devotion and dedication into taking care of your body than you do into the golf club you love so much.

In most professional sports, athletes usually reach their peak in their 20s or early 30s and retire before reaching their 40s. In some, like gymnastics and ice skating, anyone over 30 seems ancient. In golf, however, you can make a living playing professionally into your 60s and beyond. Recreationally, there's no limit to how long someone can play as long as they are fundamentally healthy. In this sense, golf is a great test of basic health. You can golf for fun past the age of 100 if your health allows it. Don't they say that anyone can golf as long as they have the strength to lift a golf club?

German golfer Bernhard Langer set the record in November 2020 as the oldest player to make the cut at the Masters Tournament. Bryson DeChambeau, a 26-year-old American professional golf icon famous for being a super-long hitter, also participated in the event. Langer was more than 700 yards behind DeChambeau in total driving distance in the final round. However, Langer finished tied for 29th at -3, while DeChambeau ended up tied for 34th at -2. How did he achieve this? Langer made up for his shorter drives by hitting more greens-in-regulation and putting better. He was 63 years old at the time. Since the age of 50, Langer has recorded some 41 wins on the PGA Champions Tour, including 11 senior majors. For many observers, what sets Langer apart is his ongoing dedication to physical fitness.

Golf is good exercise and a widely known longevity sport. It's dangerous, though, to think that means you don't need to do any other exercise. Exercise is essential not only for better health but also to play better golf. Regular strength training, good stretching for developing flexibility, and supplemental exercises for training your body in the opposite direction (where it gets less exercise) are among the most important basics of golf fitness. If you ignore such basics, not only will your golf skills fail to improve, but you won't be able to enjoy golf for as long. You'll also end up suffering from frequent injuries.

If you're under 50, you might not consider your overall health a primary factor in your golf game, but you should. If you're over 60, you're probably already aware of the effect that poor health can have on your game. The older you get, the more you'll realize that your physical condition is your golfing superpower. Start fitness training as soon as possible; the younger you are, the better. If you want to golf your whole life, you should make sure that exercise is deeply ingrained into your life, like washing your face and brushing your teeth.

Exercise for One Minute Every Hour

For us amateur golfers, it's hard to invest hours a day in fitness as the pros do, nor do we need to. It's best if you stick to a golf fitness routine of 30 minutes to an hour every day. Don't be discouraged, though, if you're busy and can't find the time to exercise. Get into the habit of moving your body whenever you get a chance in your daily life. This is called "opportunistic exercise," or "One-Minute Workouts."

One-Minute Workouts involve medium to high-intensity exercises—such as push-ups, squats, sit-ups, lunges, and planks—done to effectively use muscle strength and increase heart rate for a minute every hour. You don't necessarily have to do One-Minute Workouts for a minute. You could work out for 5 or 10 minutes. You can do this work about 10 times a day if you set your alarm to go off every hour. Think of it as doing 30 minutes of exercise divided into 10 sessions throughout the day.

Doing sets of a few different exercises when you have the time will double their effects. For example, if you do jumping jacks followed by push-ups or squats, your heart will pound, you'll be short of breath, your muscles will get pumped, and you'll sweat. In a short time you'll experience the effects of high-intensity exercise, with your heart rate, breathing, and body temperature rising and your muscles working hard. Stretching all the muscles you use for golf after such strength training exercise is even better.

It wasn't until I was in my mid-50s that I became interested in opportunistic exercise. My body wasn't what it used to be. I had black belts in taekwondo, judo, and hapkido, and my iron-like condition in my youth let me work out for hours without getting tired, but symptoms of declining energy, weaker muscle strength, and slower reflexes started to appear in middle age. This woke me up, bringing me to the realization that I would get old in no time if I left things as they were.

I was dealing with a busy schedule at the time. Since it was hard to set aside a separate time for exercise, I began moving my body whenever I got the chance. I'd put my hands on my chair, raising and lowering my body, doing dips as I read reports. I'd do push-ups, leaning against the wall above the sink before washing my hands. I'd also do what's called "bear walking"—putting my palms and soles on the floor with my butt in the air, doing a few laps around the room while crawling on all fours like a bear. In the car, at every opportunity, I'd do intestinal exercise and abdominal breathing, and I'd work on my grip and wrist strength by using a hand gripper. I developed my own way of walking, Longevity Walking, to walk in my daily life and on the golf course.

I was shocked when I visited a golf course a few months after starting to move my body like that whenever I got the chance. The number of my strokes hadn't changed significantly, but my swing was much more solid. My regret over dropping the ball into a bunker lasted only a moment; I found pleasure in thinking about how to get the ball out and onto the green, and in challenging myself to do it. Full of energy, even after a round of 18 holes, I played another round.

You might wonder how effective short bursts of exercise could be. Test it out for a week. Your body will be lighter, more agile, and energized. If you stick with it for three months, your golf swing will be more stable, and you won't get as tired on the course. The important thing is to make moving your body a habit, a part of your constitution. If you don't have a golf fitness routine yet, focus on frequency rather than duration or intensity. Your willingness may quickly decline if exercises are too intense or are a burden to you from the start.

Aim to repeat One-Minute Workouts as often as possible— but you can repeat something only once you start it, and it becomes a habit only if you repeat it. Try repeating this workout several times every day for a short time, until it becomes a habit. It's important to develop a habit of exercising regularly and consistently rather than exercising only on certain days or increasing your exercise volume. Once regular exercise becomes a habit, you can gradually increase your duration or intensity.

I recommend that you try using an approach I use whenever I feel lazy and don't want to move. I tell this to my brain every time it happens. I even say it out loud when there's no one around. "Fitness is my life. Fitness is my golf superpower and my golf lifespan." I then count "one, two, three" and jump up to start moving my body.

Move on Foot, Not in a Golf Cart

The importance of strength training for senior golfers cannot be emphasized enough. Muscle mass usually decreases gradually after the age of 30, dropping 8 percent every 10 years between the ages of 50 and 70 and by 15 percent every 10 years after that. Unless you deal with this issue, by the time you reach your 80s you will have lost about half of the muscle mass you had in your 30s.

Muscles shrink when not used. One study looked at how muscle atrophied in healthy men after they lay motionless for three weeks. The experiment showed that although the subjects' arm muscles remained the same, their leg muscles became an incredible 15 percent thinner. And the atrophied leg muscles returned to their original condition only after nine weeks of retraining.

It's also worth noting that they spent three times as much time rebuilding muscle as it took to lose the muscle. This shows how important a lifestyle of frequently moving the body is for one's health.

If you're looking for an exercise method to strengthen your leg muscles, I recommend walking and biking. On the course, if possible, move on foot instead of riding in a golf cart. The

102-year-old golfer Jongjin Lee, introduced in Part 1 of this book, was a lover of walking. He would leave his house at six o'clock every morning and walk about 5 miles on trails near his home. He walked with an umbrella whenever it rained or snowed. His cardiorespiratory function as measured in his late 90s was comparable to that of a man in his 50s. You can even achieve a meditative effect for calming the mind if you use Longevity Walking, which I'll introduce later.

Bicycling not only builds leg strength but also improves cardiorespiratory function, agility, balance, and reflexes. Since the saddle supports your weight, you can exercise for a long time without straining your joints.

I once rode a regular bicycle along the unpaved road to Sedona Mago Center in Sedona, Arizona. I didn't think it would be a big deal, since it was only a little over an hour by bicycle, but it was tough. Riding on the rough gravel road was quite a challenge. Just when I'd catch my breath, another uphill stretch would appear, making me think it would be better to carry my bicycle on my back. Since that experience, I switched to using an electric bike. Now, I can easily enjoy riding along the hilly roads of Sedona, adjusting the exercise to fit my condition.

I didn't think the workout would be that great on such a bicycle since it was motorized, but I was mistaken. The exercise effect was actually better, because now it was easy to control my breathing and the biking didn't wear me out, allowing me to ride longer and more often.

In principle, it's similar to how it's better to do an appropriate number of repetitions consistently with light dumbbells instead of overdoing it, lifting heavy weights only once in a while. I recommend an electric bike for people who want to develop leg strength but find an ordinary bicycle too much of a burden.

Exercise to Connect Your Body, Mind, and Breath

Training your body to do any complex task requires both mental and physical work. Obviously, if you can't imagine what you're trying to learn, your body will have a hard time learning it.

Many of us spend hours, days, and even months or years struggling to improve our golf game. We hit buckets of balls, pay for expensive lessons, watch countless YouTube videos, and read the latest books on the subject. But when it comes to playing an actual golf game, there's one key factor that makes all these things either useful or utterly useless. That one factor is the strength of our mind-body connection.

Have you ever been reading and suddenly realized that you can't recall anything from the last few pages? In a sense, that can happen to your body as well. There are many wrong ways to practice—approaches that won't give you much benefit. And most of them involve a problem in your mind-body connection. For example, practicing without focus, intention, and awareness—basically without mindfulness—makes it incredibly difficult to progress. The mind is an important part of practice.

Don't get this confused with being overly serious, however. We can certainly benefit from playfulness in our practice.

Actually, playfulness is a great way to increase mindfulness, not decrease it. When children play, they're highly invested in the moment. There is usually physical, mental, and emotional importance to what they're doing. As adults, however, we often "go through the motions." Our bodies are working, but our minds are stuck in unproductive patterns of judgment, avoidance, or fatigue.

Mind-body communication is a relationship that works both ways. The mind affects the body, and the body affects the mind. Let me put it like this: as your physical condition improves, you may find it easier to use your mind clearly and powerfully. Likewise, as your mental and emotional state improves, you may find it easier to train your body.

Try adding the mind-body exercises from Brain Education below to the golf fitness regimen you're already doing. Mind-body training in Brain Education is different from regular strength training and stretching. It involves using your energy sense and breathing to consciously link body and mind.

Your sense of energy combined with conscious breathing anchors the wandering mind, keeping it in the body. It's like a magnet attracting your mind to your body. The trick is to pay attention to your breathing and the sensations you feel in the moving parts of your body. For example, when doing neck exercises, focus your attention on your neck, trying to notice any changes or feelings in that area. At this time, breathe with the feeling of exhaling any old energy accumulated in your body and inhaling a fresh supply of energy. If you go with the rhythm, not rushing it, your consciousness and breathing will move together, uniting with the movements of your body.

In the next few pages, I'll introduce some mind-body exercises from Brain Education that help golfers develop muscle strength, balance, coordination, and flexibility. It's not easy to follow along just by looking at text and images, so I'm only briefly introducing the purpose and effects of each exercise and giving some tips for getting the most out of them. We've put together an Ilchi Brain Golf channel on YouTube where you can watch the techniques in detail.

Relax Your Gut to Make Your Swing Smoother

You might have heard that the gut has been called the "second brain" because of how much it influences our overall condition, including the state of our "first brain." Gut health affects everything from the obvious (the quality of your digestion) to the incredible (emotions and mental health). Balance, breathing, blood pressure, flexibility, coordination, and energy levels are just a few of the health aspects that may be affected by your gut. To make a long story short, if you want to upgrade your overall condition, you can't go wrong by taking care of your gut.

For many people, "gut health" conjures up images of restrictive diets, probiotics, and herbal supplements. While these can be extremely helpful to some people, I'm going to recommend something much simpler: exercise your gut. I don't just mean your core muscles, although that's an added benefit of what I'm proposing. I mean to actively move your abdominal muscles so that your internal organs become less stiff.

If you think about it, it makes sense that our intestines should be strong, flexible, and active. They do a lot of work digesting food, and any blockage or stiffness in the abdomen is typically going to make you very uncomfortable. Any exercise, from walking to swimming to deep breathing, can help to activate this part of your body. But to get the most bang for your buck, try moving the abdominal muscles themselves in and out. By doing so, you'll be able to release tension, increase circulation, and naturally deepen your breath.

Concentrate on your lower abdomen, repeatedly pulling it in and pushing it out. When pulling your belly in, suck it in as deeply as possible, as if trying to touch your back with your navel. You should also contract and tighten your anus at this time. When you push your belly out, push gently enough to feel the pressure in your abdomen as if you are blowing air into a balloon. Start with about 50 repetitions, gradually increasing this to 300 or more when you get used to the

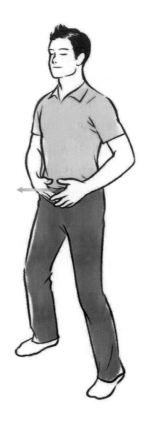

exercise. It's possible to do about 100 repetitions per minute, so once you're used to it, it's not too hard to do 1,000 repetitions over 10 minutes, working continuously. Doing 1,000 repetitions a day heats your belly, creating the condition of Water Up, Fire Down—the "cool head and warm belly" described in the previous section of this book.

What benefits can you expect to see on the golf course after doing intestinal exercise?

First, you'll have better flexibility. You'll be amazed at how much the condition of your abdomen affects your ability to stretch, rotate, and swing. Your legs may feel stronger, your back looser, and your arms freer.

Second, you can enjoy greater strength. A free and flexible core allows the body to move efficiently and with power instead of fighting against itself. If you've ever tried playing a sport after eating a big meal, you've probably noticed how much slower and heavier your body feels. Intestinal exercise can help you feel light and strong.

Third, you'll have deeper breathing. The benefits of breathing are well known but are often overlooked in the course of day-to-day golf. Breathing can help you stay more relaxed, focused, and energized on the golf course—and we all know how much of a difference that mindset can bring to our game.

Fourth, you'll develop better balance. The combination of flexibility, strength, relaxation, and easy movement can help you feel more balanced in your swing.

Finally, you'll feel less fatigue and discomfort. Over the course of a round, do you see the quality of your play suffer as your body and mind begin to tire? Does your body feel achy after a round of golf? Intestinal exercise can help keep your body feeling healthier and more supple even after playing 18 or 36 holes.

You can do intestinal exercise either sitting or lying down. You can also do this practice while driving to and from work. It's perfect for when you're stopped at a traffic light waiting for the signal to change. In South Korea, it often takes an hour or two to drive to a golf course. Doing intestinal exercise calms your mind and is an excellent warm-up on your way to play golf, and it helps you recover from fatigue on your way home.

Strengthen Your Core with the Monkey Pose

It might seem counterintuitive, but holding your body still can actually be one of the best ways to strengthen your muscles and joints. In particular, isometric exercise (contracting muscles while in a static position) can make a huge difference in your overall wellness by helping to align, strengthen, and even relax your body. If you've ever tried a "wall sit," you know how challenging it can be.

The monkey pose is a core-strengthening exercise in which you balance on your tailbone with your arms and legs held up in the air with knees bent. It's a challenging exercise. You can modify it by keeping your heels on the floor and adjusting the angle of your spine and the bend of your knees.

This kind of exercise is best done after a good warm-up and perhaps some stretching. The real magic happens when you focus internally on your breathing while holding an isometric pose. In the monkey posture, while balancing on

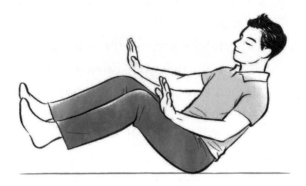

your tailbone, focus on the elongation of your spine and the depth of your breath. As you breathe slowly and smoothly, you are actually strengthening the internal muscles related to your breathing. Without getting deep into anatomical explanations, activating the core muscles to hold this posture acts as a counter pressure to the internal muscles related to breathing, giving them something to push against. This unique combination results in a sense of energy in the core and a general feeling of strength and centeredness.

Power, balance, and coordination all depend on having a clear awareness of the body's center of gravity. For many of us, this awareness is dulled because of stiffness or weakness in the spine, hips, and abdomen, related to excess tension in the chest, neck, and shoulders. No matter how much you practice your golf swing, unless you release accumulated tension and develop strength and awareness of your core, there will be a limit to how far you can progress in developing it.

The 100-Year Golfer

The great thing about the monkey posture is that anyone, regardless of their age or condition, can give it a try, modifying it as needed. Whether they hold the posture for only 10 seconds by lifting their legs while sitting in an armchair or challenge themselves to hold it for three or four minutes without touching the ground, anyone can improve their strength and deepen their breathing.

Try holding the monkey posture every other day. Start out by checking your stamina. Don't overdo it; the goal isn't to make your abdominal muscles sore for a week. You should be able to breathe throughout the exercise. Once you know your limit, make a plan to increase your staying power each time you practice. If you focus on using your breath and concentrating, you should notice that you're increasing the time you can spend in this posture a little more each time.

On the golf course, you may notice benefits related to a stronger core and more energy. With continued practice, this posture can help align your body to avoid excess stress or tension that might otherwise accumulate over time from performing repetitive motions.

Develop Balance and Flexibility with Plate Balancing

At its best, swinging a golf club feels like an effortless dance, with natural rhythm and power. For most of us, however, this feeling is rare. More often than not, we may be aware of excess torque and tension as we attempt to incorporate a new technique or overcome mental stress. In addition, the vast majority of us swing in only one direction, day after day, so we develop imbalances in our musculature and body alignment to match.

If you've ever tried tai chi, you may have noticed that learning a new series of movements can be complicated. Adding another element, such as holding a golf club, challenges your awareness even more. If you want to develop your balance, body awareness, and coordination, I suggest that you start by setting the clubs aside and picking up something else: a plate.

Actually, you can start without holding anything at all in your hands. Simply assume the proper stance and imagine holding something in your hand as you rotate it through the "plate balancing" infinity motion.

As you move through this exercise (as shown on the Ilchi Brain Golf channel on YouTube), you'll become aware of how your body flows. Because plate balancing is basically tracing a figure 8 in the air, there's no need to consider a beginning or an end. You can simply enter into a kind of moving meditation. This exercise works the wrists, elbows, shoulders, spine, hips, and knees in a coordinated manner, so you'll be training your body to move smoothly and efficiently, and with purpose. Let go of any need to finish the exercise and simply give yourself over to the flow of the movement. There's no point in trying to go faster or harder; instead, your aim can be to feel more balanced, more flexible, more aware of how your body is working.

Try plate balancing for three to five minutes each day. (You can do more if you'd like.) You should notice added functional flexibility and strength after practicing. Best of all, you can practice on both sides of your body. At first, you may see differences in the strength and flexibility of your left and right sides. This is a great chance to take stock of your overall body balance and resolve any imbalances.

A balanced and coordinated body makes you much more likely to remain strong and healthy over time. And you may notice that swinging a club feels easier and that you have more strength after doing plate balancing because your various joints and muscles are now working in harmony.

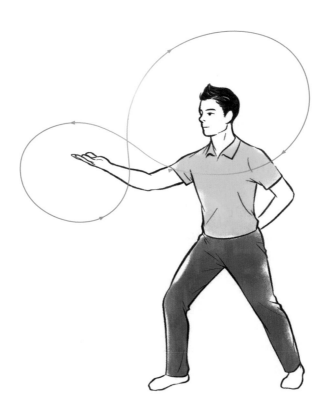

Develop Rhythm and Coordination with Free Dance

Proprioception—the ability to sense where your body is in space—is one of golf's most important and challenging aspects. By now, most of us who enjoy golf have seen countless hours of professional golfers swinging clubs. In our heads, we know what the golf swing is supposed to look like, and we imagine ourselves swinging in the same way. But the way your swing feels to you is not necessarily the way it looks to others. Or, to put it more bluntly—your swing isn't as pretty as you think it is.

This isn't something to get upset about. Crafting a beautiful golf swing takes years, if not decades, for even the most talented players. The real question is whether you're able to create new movements when you want to.

Have you ever taken a lesson or watched a video and realized, "I think I need to do more of that," but when you try, it's difficult to do anything other than what you've done before? Many golfers know their swing faults, but they aren't able to work creatively to change them. Applying a new element to their swing seems to make the whole thing fall apart.

Even the best players in the world struggle to adjust to new techniques or swing thoughts. What separates those who can adapt from those who can't is something I like to call "imaginative movement." Suppose you want to change the way you do things. You have to move your body in new and unusual ways without panicking or losing awareness. At first it'll feel strange and even counterproductive. Being able to navigate this period of change is a matter of having a strong and healthy mind-body connection. In other words, you need to enjoy the discomfort of the change process.

Free dance is one of the best ways I know to help develop this quality. Free dance is all about rhythm, feeling, and fun. There are no rules, judgments, or requirements other than moving your body to the music. Free dance is most certainly not about looking good in the eyes of an audience. If this is your concern when you hear the word "dance," I want you to practice by yourself. Make the phrase, "Dance like nobody's watching," literally true for you.

If you find the idea of dancing by yourself boring or a waste of time, I encourage you to focus more deeply on your own body sense. Which parts of your body feel heavy? Which areas feel light? Do you enjoy one kind of movement more than another? Do different songs naturally make you want to move in different ways? There are no right or wrong answers to these questions. They are all about connecting with yourself, with your mind and body.

If you enjoy and practice free dance regularly, you may notice that you can incorporate new golf swing techniques more quickly and easily because now your body and mind don't resist change. Beyond that, you can deepen your sense of rhythm, balance, and leverage through free dance.

I like dancing, and I dance often. These days, my favorite dance songs are BTS' "Dynamite" and "My Universe," which they did with Coldplay. They've graduated now, but BTS members were students of Global Cyber University, where I serve as president. Dancing to BTS songs improves my mood, thanks to their bright, young, uplifting energy—and it makes me expect good things from tomorrow's round of golf!

Tap Your Toes to Relax Your Tired Brain and Muscles

At some point, if you've practiced golf long enough, you've probably realized that you play your best when you get out of your own way. What does this mean? For many of us, overanalyzing our swing can become our biggest problem.

When you're playing well, you might describe it as being "in the zone" or "in a flow state." What it is not is "being in your head."

In our modern world, we are constantly being stimulated to think. Our brains are bombarded with information requiring an interpretation and a reaction from us. Eventually, this "head-centered" way of life can become a physiological habit. Getting "out of your head" can be almost impossible. I want to recommend a very simple exercise to help you do that. It's not going to be something you do on the golf course. This is for your day-to-day life, and it's called toe tapping.

Toe tapping is an easy motion, but it has a variety of effects. It reduces inflammation in the feet and legs by promoting blood circulation, makes the hip joints flexible, and relieves fatigue. I recommend that you do it before going to bed, since its relaxing effect is powerful enough to slow your brain waves and put you into a state of semi-sleep. If you go to bed after doing toe tapping on the night before you play a round of golf, you can get deep, restful sleep. On days when you've played a round, this practice helps you relax your weary brain and muscles and recharge your energy.

Lie comfortably with your back on the floor. Spread your arms to your sides slightly away from your body, and open your hands, palms facing up. With your legs touching, tap the insides of your feet together to make a rapping sound. Move your feet quickly, alternating between your big toes touching each other and your little toes barely touching the floor.

Now, as you exhale through your mouth, imagine the stress and tired energy leaving your body through your outgoing breath. It should feel as though you're cleaning the energy in your body, like turning on a fan and blowing stagnant air out of a room.

Do about 50 to 100 repetitions of toe tapping, and then stop and breathe comfortably for about a minute, imagining the stagnant energy leaving your body through your toes. It's good to do 300 to 500 repetitions once you're comfortable with the exercise. If that's difficult, you can take a break in the middle. Practice toe tapping at least once a day, perhaps before going to bed.

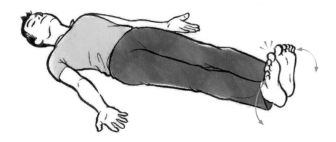

Exercise Your Joints to Build Strength

If you want to feel your body's strength return quickly, I recommend joint relaxation and strengthening exercises.

Many people suffer from stiff joints. If your knees are stiff, it doesn't matter how strong your quads are; you're going to have a tough time feeling like you can go up a few flights of stairs. If your back and shoulders are stiff, you're not going to want to carry boxes to the car. Basically, stiff joints make it difficult to use your natural muscle strength.

By loosening up and exercising your joints, you should notice a feeling of greater strength and mobility in your arms, legs, and back. To accomplish this, I recommend joint rotation exercises. You might have seen some of these practices in martial arts and dance classes. Rotating your joints stimulates blood flow and energy awareness without straining muscles and ligaments. You'll also mobilize the synovial fluid that lubricates joints.

Especially in golf, it's not so much the big muscles that limit our speed, balance, and control; they're limited by the small, stabilizing muscles and joint connections becoming stiff. Traditional exercises working large muscle groups, while generally beneficial, may not target these crucial areas. But rotating the joints is a great way to strengthen them. Through rotation, you can relax and strengthen your joints without straining your muscles and ligaments. You can ensure that blood circulates through every corner of your joints while also promoting the movement of joint fluid.

Rotate the joints of your neck, shoulders, wrists, lower back, knees, and ankles 5 to 10 times in one direction, then the same number of times in the opposite direction. Breathe comfortably with your mouth open slightly, with long exhalations. If you maintain your energy sense while doing joint rotations, your joints will relax, allowing you to feel tension being released and energy filling your joints.

Even if your large muscles are well developed—those of your shoulders, back, arms, and legs—stiff joints will limit the speed, balance, and control of your swing. Senior golfers in particular should be meticulous about their golf fitness and make sure to include joint exercises. Whatever age you are now, if you want to golf until you're 100, the time will come when you have to make joint health a top priority.

Developing Flexibility Took Six Strokes off My Game

By Gerald Martori
64-year-old man, New York, USA, 50 years of golf experience

It's been close to 50 years since I learned to golf when I was a teenager, thanks to the influence of my father, who was a golfer. I've always liked golf, but I barely played four or five rounds a year after getting married and having children. I worked as a high school principal until I retired four years ago. Since then, I've been enjoying golf about twice a week.

When you get older, you have to do something to develop flexibility. In my experience, nothing beats the plate balancing I learned at the Body & Brain Yoga center. I was never a yoga guy. My wife got me into it when I was working. The practice helped me deal with the stress of work and become more flexible.

Plate balancing deeply stretches the lower back, upper back, shoulders, arms, and sides and develops a sense of balance. I can hear my body cracking, popping, and stretching while doing the exercise. Whenever I move my shoulders while doing plate balancing, I think it's really similar to the shoulder turn of a golf swing.

I started running when I was young, and I'm still doing it now, but before Body & Brain practice, I never felt that my body was flexible. Now, when I stand and bend over, my hands touch the floor. We've got a dedicated space in the attic: the "Zen Den." There I regularly exercise, training my core, hips, and back as well as my flexibility. Thanks to the flexibility I've developed through this training, I've taken 6 to 10 strokes off my game. My handicap is around 11 to 20.

One thing I've been concentrating on is meditation. I try to remain in the moment while golfing or doing other exercises, focusing on the task at hand. With golf, it's shot to shot. Beautiful drive and then a duck-hook into the water. I just hit a great one, and now I can't do it. It's about refocusing on that particular shot at the moment and not thinking about the next one or the last one. Most golfers will hit a bad shot and curse. You'll see that pros can hit a bad shot and recover. I'm sure they're mad, but they focus back on the task at hand.

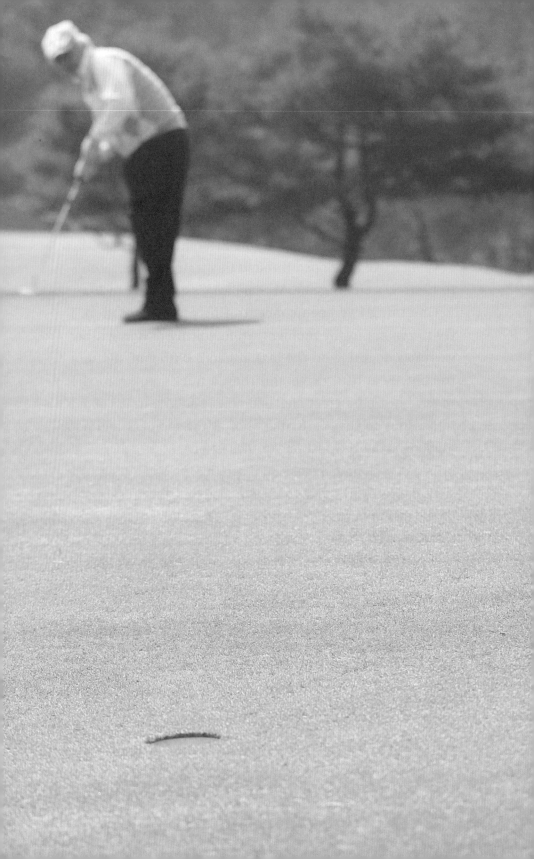

THIRD ART: BREATHING

Develop Your Golf Mentality with Breathing

My Breathing Stopped
after I Fell from a Horse

It was a summer day 13 years ago, and I was riding a horse near Sedona Mago Center in Sedona, Arizona. I'd been riding regularly for nearly 10 years, and horseback riding in the Arizona high desert was like a walk in the park. I was immersed in thought as I sat in the saddle.

My horse, Su, was plodding along a path lined with prickly pears and groves of low junipers. Su was my favorite horse—smart, kind, and curious. Having long ridden together, we understood each other simply by the looks in our eyes. But then, suddenly surprised by something, Su reared on his hind legs and then started galloping. Having let go of the reins, I bent over and clung to his back as he raced along. The instant I thought I'd finally gotten hold of the reins, Su suddenly jerked to a stop from a full gallop and started shaking. The force of that stop instantly sent me flying from his back.

My body soared through the air as I was thrown to the ground. The martial arts falling techniques I'd done in my youth were ingrained in my body, causing me to rotate about 15 degrees in midair without even realizing it. Thanks to that twist, my buttocks hit the ground first instead of my head. But I was thrown with such force that the impact was severe. My lower back cracked loudly, and the taste of blood rose inside my mouth.

I could hear people running from afar, calling me in shock. I tried wiggling my hands and feet, and fortunately, they moved, but the pain was so bad that I cried out—"Agh!" And my breathing had stopped. I wasn't inhaling or exhaling. It was as if I'd forgotten how to breathe. Suddenly, I thought I might die. I was lying on the ground, unable to move or breathe, when the sky unexpectedly caught my eye. It was so beautiful! There I was, with pain surging through my body and thoughts of impending death rising in my mind, observing that the sky was beautiful. The human brain is truly a fantastic thing.

Looking up at the deep blue sky, I felt like it was about to suck me in. I'll be able to breathe if heaven wants to save me, I thought. If not, this will be the last sky I see. I felt my mind growing calm. I tried exhaling very slowly, and luckily, I felt the breath leaving my body. And I breathed in. I was so grateful then for that precious gulp of air I took into my lungs. The wavering flame of my life seemed to blaze as my body started to breathe again.

The time when I wasn't breathing, at most a minute or so, felt like an eternity. Before that accident, I had developed and taught various breathing methods for close to 30 years. Still, my experience that day made me feel with my whole body that breathing is life.

It took me two months to recover after falling from that horse. Unable to move my body properly, I could do two things: vibrate my body, moving it minutely from side to side, and breathe. I spoke with my body through breathing, and I was able to recover as rapidly as I did—surprising my doctors—because my body assisted in its own healing.

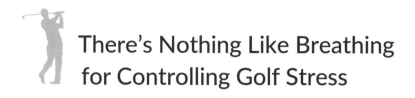

There's Nothing Like Breathing for Controlling Golf Stress

How does stress affect your golf game over the course of a round? Most of us feel first-tee jitters, even the pros. But stress is more than just a reaction to the pressure of hitting your first shot or playing in front of a crowd. Stress can come from a missed shot, a rushed putt, someone's inconsiderate action during a round, even from your own expectations. Stress makes you stiff and distracted. Later it can leave you feeling drained and unmotivated.

Some people seem to thrive under pressure. They react to stress by focusing more intensely, which appears to strengthen them. Others crumble under pressure. How about you? Probably you've experienced both phenomena.

In golf, as in life, we can't avoid stress. If you want to play, you must expect stress. The difference between wilting versus thriving is in how we react to stressful situations. Do we lose our cool and start following a cascade of negative feelings and thoughts? Or do we channel our stress energy into controlled and productive processes? I want to share something that has helped me deal with stress, both on the golf course and in life: breathing.

How is your breathing on the course? If your answer is "I don't know," you're not alone. Most of us spend little to no time focusing on our breath. After all, it happens whether we pay attention or not. But does it really? Of course, you'll keep breathing, even when you're asleep. But the quality and effect of your breath can be quite different depending on your awareness, especially under stress.

Breathing is like a shield when you're under attack from stress. Or it's like aikido, a martial art that focuses not on blocking but on redirecting an attacker's energy to throw them off balance. Breathing can help you redirect the energy of anxiety or frustration into productive avenues.

Why is breathing so powerful? The autonomic nervous system regulates the critical vital phenomena of our bodies, such as pulse, blood pressure, temperature, and respiration. These functions happen spontaneously, whether we're aware of them or not. But what makes breathing different from other vital functions is that it can be consciously controlled. You cannot intentionally raise or lower your blood pressure or body temperature directly, but you can make your breathing slower or faster. By consciously controlling your respiration, you can alleviate the stress response occurring in your autonomic nervous system and positively affect your other vitals, such as pulse and blood pressure.

Have you ever measured how many breaths you take per minute? If not, give it a try now. The normal breathing rate for an adult at rest is 10 to 15 breaths per minute. What would happen if you cut your usual rate in half? Even lowering it to less than 10 breaths per minute will make your mind feel more relaxed. The ideal rhythm is a breath every 12 seconds so that you breathe five times in a minute. Consciously controlling respiration to breathe at this rate increases cardiorespiratory efficiency and provides a surprising sense of groundedness.

Is breathing going to help you hit your drive right down the middle on the first tee? I can't promise that. I still suffer from first-tee jitters from time to time, and I've been meditating for more than 40 years. Look at it this way: are you better off when you take a few deep breaths before hitting your first shot? Almost undoubtedly, the answer is yes. But how should you breathe?

Three-Step Breathing for Golfers

I'm going to share three simple steps for better breathing that you can take onto the golf course.

The first step is to relax your shoulders and chest because this is where much of our stress and tension is held, and these areas are relatively easier to relax than some of the deeper parts of the body. So, start with a couple of deep breaths, exhaling through the mouth. In Eastern traditions, we say that the mouth is like a giant acupressure point. Lots of energy enters and leaves the body through the mouth. Before going deeper, begin by using this breathing technique to relax your shoulders and chest.

Breathe in through your nose for three or four seconds; if you're feeling significant stress, two or three seconds is long enough. If you can, hold your breath for a comfortable moment, feeling the expansion of your chest. Then exhale as smoothly as you can through your mouth. Again, if you're feeling significant stress, it may come out as a whoosh of air—but that's okay. If possible, lengthen your exhalation to four to six seconds, and feel your rib cage relaxing. Repeat this breathing four or five times if you can, lengthening your exhalation a little more each time. Focus on the center of your chest, and imagine warm energy melting away any tension you are holding there.

Here's an additional technique you can use to make this breathing practice more effective. It's called "body tapping," and it involves gently stimulating acupressure points related to the heart and lungs. With your fingertips or loose fists, tap the areas below your collarbones on each side of your chest. You can use both hands at once or alternate between them. Breathe out through your mouth while tapping. If you watch closely as PGA tour players wait for their turn to tee off, you might catch a glimpse of some of them using a simple sequence of body tapping called emotional freedom technique (EFT) to relax and focus.

After tapping for 10 or 20 seconds, stop to feel the effects. You might notice that your breathing is now deeper and smoother, and that you feel slightly more relaxed. If you're in a high-stress situation, though, don't be surprised if it's hard to notice any change. Like many other aspects of dealing with stress on the course, trusting your routine is most important.

Now that you've started to relax your chest and shoulders, you're ready to go deeper. The next area to focus on is your solar plexus, or stomach area.

Inhale through your nose for three or four seconds and gently exhale through your mouth for four to six seconds. Focus on relaxing your upper-abdominal muscles. This might be an unusual thing to feel. If you tend to hold your tension near your stomach (think butterflies in the stomach), you might notice more tension before you sense any relaxation. Keep going, imagining your stomach getting softer and lighter.

As with most things that involve mind and body coordination, relaxation breathing techniques become more effective the more you practice. Try these techniques at home when you're not under stress, and you'll find them working better the next time you're on the course or in any stressful life situation, such as giving a lecture, resolving an argument, driving in traffic, or taking a test.

Step three is where the magic really happens because it activates our main energy center. In Korean, we call this center the *"dahnjon,"* and it's located 1 or 2 inches below the navel and 2 or 3 inches inside the body. If you've heard of "abdominal breathing," then you'll have some idea of the importance of deep breathing to stimulate this area. By focusing specifically on this dahnjon area, you may tap into something beyond relaxation. With practice, you can feel a precise and powerful sense of your center.

Breathe using the method introduced in the previous steps. If possible, breathe in and out only through your nose, without using your mouth. Concentrating your awareness in your lower abdomen, slowly inhale while pushing your belly out. Pause until you feel a sense of fullness, and then exhale until you get the feeling that your lower abdomen is being pulled in. Hold your breath only to a comfortable degree— not until your chest is tight and your face turns red. Slowly and rhythmically repeat the movements of pushing out your lower abdomen as you inhale and pulling it in as you exhale. At a pace that is comfortable for you, push and pull your lower abdomen consistently and rhythmically.

Your inhalations and exhalations continue naturally when your body and mind are comfortable. You automatically exhale when you've breathed in enough, and you automatically inhale once you've breathed out enough. Once you've mastered your sense of energy, your lower abdomen will grow warmer, and you'll get a pleasant feeling of fullness as energy accumulates in your dahnjon as you breathe.

When doing the three-step breathing described above, beginners can place their hands on their chest, upper abdomen, and lower abdomen, respectively. Feeling through your hands the rhythm of each body part rising and falling with your breath will help you concentrate.

Chest breathing and upper abdominal breathing are good for relaxing the body and mind and releasing tension and anxiety on the golf course. Dahnjon breathing, which focuses on the belly, not only helps with relaxation, but helps build a powerful center in the lower abdomen with regular practice. Not only will this technique help you feel more relaxed and focused, but it can also become a source of power and balance during your swing.

Breathing in Threes: Three In, Three Out

This next breathing method is good for when you're waiting your turn to tee off or moving between holes on the golf course. At holes where your game isn't going well, it's easy to get irritated and let your mind fill with thoughts about how you stupidly hit the ball in a water hazard or absurdly missed a 2-foot putt. When that happens, try this way of breathing.

Inhale three times and exhale three times. This lets you take in and let out more air than when you breathe once each way. I base this on my own experience of exhaling very slowly, several times, bit by bit, when my breathing had stopped after I was thrown from my horse.

Inhale, feeling yourself filling your lungs with air, once, twice, three times. Then hold it, concentrating on the feeling of your chest expanding. When you exhale, breathe the air out of your lungs completely, over three outgoing breaths. Feel full when you inhale, refreshed when you exhale. Repeating this just 5 to 10 times slows your brain waves and brings mental stability.

Breathe for Five Minutes in Sleeping Tiger Pose

If you'd like to work on upgrading your breathing when you're not on the course, I have a powerful exercise called "sleeping tiger." This simple breathing technique strengthens the breathing muscles and core muscles. It helps you clear your mind, increase your focus, and warm your dahnjon energy center.

Sleeping tiger is best practiced in a quiet, comfortable space so that you can bring your focus inside yourself. Preferably, find a soft but firm surface, such as a thick mat or carpeted floor, for this exercise. Lying on your back, lift your arms and legs up with your knees bent. Your feet should be slightly above knee level, ankles flexed slightly so your toes are pulled toward you. Your elbows should be subtly bent, with your palms facing the ceiling in line with your chest. You don't want to bring them up over your head. The key point is to keep your lower back pressed against the floor. This will ensure that you activate your core muscles and protect your spine, and it should allow you to focus your mind on your lower abdomen.

This exercise is uniquely beneficial because it requires not only physical strength but also mental focus. The sleeping tiger position is physically harder to hold the more distracted you are. Those who practice this posture regularly learn the importance of breathing, core energy, and awareness for physical performance.

When you're holding the sleeping tiger posture, you're training yourself to release unnecessary tension and activate the stabilizing core muscles. Beginners may notice their bodies becoming tense—a natural reaction as the big muscles of the legs, back, and shoulders try to hold the posture. Most people will reach their limit in three to five minutes. To hold the pose longer, you'll need to learn how to relax your big muscles consciously and to rely instead on your breathing and the deeper stabilizing muscles. For many of us, a sedentary lifestyle has weakened these stabilizing muscles. Inflexibility in the hips, shoulders, and back also adds to muscle tension and instability.

Aim to hold sleeping tiger for five minutes if you can, and see how it goes. If your muscles are very strong, you may not notice much. Keep going. At some point, you'll feel vibrations starting in your legs, back, and arms. This means the big muscles are tiring and your stabilizing and breathing muscles are about to get their chance to wake up. Focus on relaxing and breathing, putting all your energy into keeping your lower back comfortably against the floor.

If you practice sleeping tiger regularly, you should notice a new sense of your center. Physically, you may feel stronger and more relaxed. Your balance should feel more stable, and your breathing will naturally be deeper. How does this translate to the golf course? You will notice that your swing is smoother and more balanced, producing more speed, power, and—hopefully—control. One of the major differences between the tour pros we watch on TV and us average players is swing stability. If you're going to get the clubhead moving at 120 miles per hour, your balance needs to be extremely good. Otherwise, hitting a straight shot is virtually impossible. Even the pros struggle with this, obviously.

Sleeping tiger, as you'll find out, will challenge you mentally as much as it will physically. As you hold the posture, you'll notice your mind wanting to escape or adjust in order to make things more comfortable. But if you allow your mind to wander, you'll find the posture increasingly impossible to hold. Only by maintaining your focus despite the challenge will your body be able to stay in sleeping tiger.

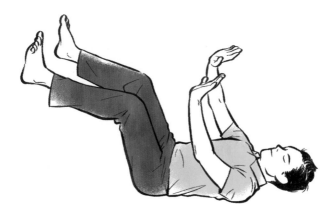

The physical benefits of doing this exercise will improve your golf game, but I believe the mental benefits will be even greater. How often do most of us unconsciously try to escape from stress rather than face it with power? In fact, the training that you'll do with your body will strengthen your willpower as well. You'll be able to meet stress with confidence and concentration because your mind is like a muscle. It gets stronger when you challenge it in a healthy way.

Fine-Tune and Take Care of Your Life with Conscious Breathing

The most important thing in all the breathing methods I've introduced is to breathe "consciously." Normally your brain keeps you breathing, but now you're giving your brain a signal, saying, "I'm doing the breathing." You're breathing consciously, not just letting it happen automatically. Aim to breathe with devotion in each breath. Get the feeling that you're giving the kiss of life to yourself. Try to do your best, imagining that your body won't breathe unless you breathe for it, unless you breathe consciously.

Breathing is the highest act of love for your body. Through breathing you can interact with yourself, control your emotions, and give yourself confidence. Many breathing methods can help your golf game; there's no single best technique. The best breathing method is the one that works for you. Find through your own body the approach that's best suited for you.

Get the feeling that you're fine-tuning and caring for your life through your breathing. As you inhale and exhale, feel gratitude for nature, which sustains our lives without asking for anything in return. The more time you spend breathing consciously, the more your composure will increase and the more your consideration for others and your care for nature will grow on the golf course.

Learning How to Accept Failure through Breathing

By Courtney Lindop
35-year-old woman, Boston, USA, three years of golf experience

My parents are from Scotland, so growing up, golfing was always around. But it wasn't until I started practicing Brain Education with Body & Brain Yoga that I felt the desire to play myself. The truth is, I had suffered from anxiety and depression when I was young, and the thought of playing sports was overwhelming.

My parents always encouraged me to play golf socially, but I would reject their invitations for one reason or another. It wasn't until I developed a stronger awareness of how to deal with nervousness and negative thoughts through Brain Education that I could actually imagine that golf might be fun.

Part of dealing with anxiety and depression was being very sensitive to failure. Golf, as we all know, is full of failure. In the past, I wouldn't have had the patience to deal with failure long enough to get to the good part. I would have given up too quickly and missed the fun.

Now, using breathing techniques, I am able to embrace the ups and downs of golf and still enjoy the game. Best of all, I see myself improving in a way that gives me hope and confidence. If I can see progress in my golf game, I know I can apply the same work ethic to anything in my life and see results. I consider that a different kind of consciousness. It feels like a different way of living.

You could say that Brain Education techniques give me some space to watch my emotions instead of reacting to them. That little bit of space is the difference between being irritated at a mistake and then moving on, versus starting a downward spiral of negative thinking. I think everyone, from beginner to pro, could probably benefit from this practice.

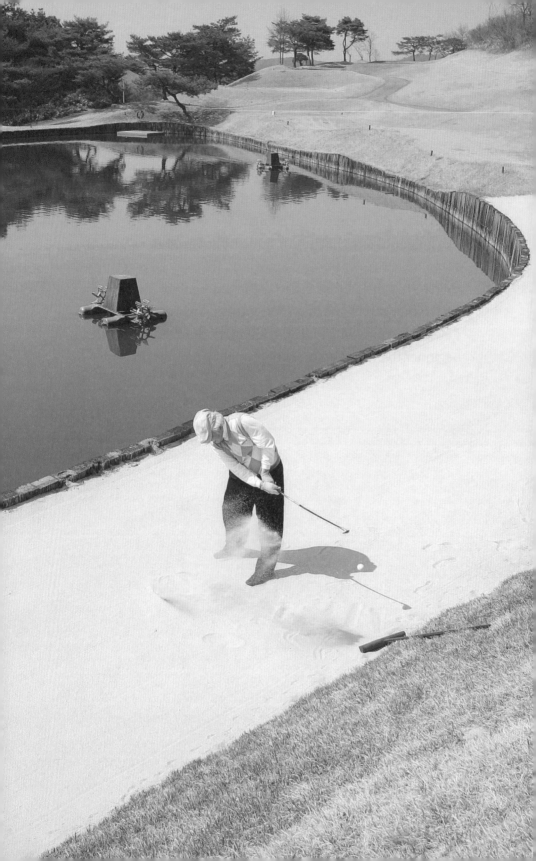

Get into the Zone with Relaxed Concentration

Make Your Entire Golf Experience a Meditation

When I lecture about meditation, the first thing I try to share with people is that meditation can be anything. You don't have to be sitting cross-legged on the floor or humming a mantra, although those are both effective meditation techniques. Fundamentally, meditation is about establishing inward attention and minimizing the effects of outward distraction.

Here's another insight: quieting outward distraction doesn't mean being blind to the world around you. In fact, when you meditate and focus inward, you might notice that you see the world around you more clearly. You can feel things as they are instead of through the filter of random thoughts and emotions.

In a sense, anything that allows you to deepen your inner awareness beyond thoughts and emotions can be meditation. For some people, that might be a hobby—perhaps woodworking, photography, or poetry writing. For others, it might be a physical activity such as cross-country skiing, swimming, or even archery, running, or martial arts. Or, of course, golf.

Have you ever reached a meditative state while golfing? If so, what did it feel like to you? I believe that part of the attraction for many of us golf fanatics is the entrance this sport provides into different states of consciousness.

When I say "different consciousness," I'm simply referring to different patterns of awareness. I'm sure you've felt it: you sense and see things differently on different days. Maybe you head to the golf course after finishing a long and stressful project and notice that your mind is more peaceful and relaxed than usual, and your golf game suddenly feels stable and natural. Maybe when you've been irritated by something at home, or when you're worried about an upcoming event, you notice that your game has become scattered and unpredictable. More than just moods, these are different states of consciousness, and they affect every aspect of your life: mind, body, and spirit.

When you achieve that state of relaxed concentration, you're not just feeling good. In fact, your energy changes, affecting the way your brain and body are working. You can feel that your brain is calm and clear, your decision-making is reasonable and relaxed, your body feels light and strong, and your emotions are flowing naturally and harmoniously, even when you face obstacles or make mistakes. Don't you want to play golf in this "zone" more often?

Being "in the zone" is a well-known phenomenon among athletes, artists, musicians, and performers. It means you've reached a flow state in which thought, action, and feeling harmonize to produce optimal results. In a sense, getting in the zone is a kind of meditation, often achieved through music or movement, in which you're filled with a clear sense of purpose and a feeling of creative expression.

Golf is perhaps the ultimate in-the-zone sport. It's just you, the club, the ball, and the environment. In a sense, golf is the ultimate practice for getting in the zone because the primary challenge isn't overcoming an opponent but mastering your own mind and body.

I'm going to introduce a few functional meditations for helping you deepen your immersion, maintain your composure, and develop your concentration on the golf course. But I want to encourage you to turn your entire golf experience into meditation. No special skills are required for this. All you have to do is shine the light of your awareness on your golf experience.

Most of the time, meditation isn't about having no thoughts. Instead, you can think of meditation as the practice of separating awareness from thoughts. Yes, the thoughts will still be there, but your awareness doesn't have to react to each one. Meditation is observing life phenomena and experiences just as they are, without the filters of thoughts, emotions, or ideas. It's about shining the light of your awareness on your breathing, eating, sleeping, and defecating, on your working and playing, thinking and feeling, speaking and doing, and on your habits.

Whether it's to relieve your tension and anxiety on the first tee or to keep your composure in the face of mistakes and challenges on the course, no matter what meditative practice you use, meditation is ultimately about harnessing the power of self-awareness.

Your Brain Is the Best Golf Coach

Great athletes and musicians improve their performances through a cycle of anticipation-observation-reflection, sometimes raising their performance to the level of art. If we apply this same cycle to golf, our entire experience of the game can become a powerful meditation.

Before a game, anticipate your performance by meditating on the question "How will I play the next round?" Visualize the swing you'll use and the day's golf game in your imagination. Vividly imagine your golf swings, gestures, and even feelings. Preparing your brain in advance reduces fear and tension and helps you stand eager and confident on the tee.

After you've prepared in this way, your attitude during the actual round of golf should be one of observation. You're both a performer and an observer. The question to keep in mind at this time is, "What am I doing?" Without any judgment about doing well or doing poorly, observe with close attention and an open mind what you're doing and what's happening. Take 10 seconds before every tee shot to focus not only on how you're golfing, but also on how you're behaving. Are you maintaining equanimity, or have you been reacting? Can you remember your intention from before the round?

Take time to reflectively replay your game after you finish your round. Professional players of Go, a board game that requires a great deal of strategizing and intuition to master, usually replay a game after they finish it, regardless of whether they've won or lost. They replay the entire game by themselves, playing both their own role and their opponent's. Through this process, they gain insight into moves they hadn't seen before, and that insight becomes a source of wisdom for making better choices in the next game.

Many golfers have an intense desire to talk about their round after finishing. It's a common joke that every golfer wants to tell you about how they should have scored better and would have if not for a few simple mistakes. Talking to your friends may release some of your anguish, but doing a reflective play by yourself will give you more insights.

On days when you've finished a round, sit down and replay the game in your imagination while asking yourself, "Could I have done it some other way?" Then when you practice, try applying the realizations or insights you've gained. One hour of practice when the memories of your round are fresh can be more valuable than 10 hours of ordinary practice. This is why so many professionals go straight to the practice range after finishing a tournament round. To make this work, you need an open mind that lets you see novel things—not a mind closed by self-recrimination, regret, or preconceived judgments.

Imagine someone who practices anticipation-observation-reflection every time they play a round, and someone else who spends the time before a game anxiously fidgeting, then plays the game distracted and not knowing what they're doing, and afterward just wants to forget and never think about it again. Suppose these two have both golfed for a decade. How much of a difference would there be between them?

Applying the cycle of anticipation-observation-reflection can turn your entire golf experience into a wonderful meditation. By doing this, you'll be able to use both contemplative and creative meditation. Contemplative meditation is about calming your thoughts and emotions, observing the mind attentively, and bringing awareness to what's really happening in the present moment. Creative meditation, as the words suggest, is done to gain the insight, inspiration, and confidence to create new things. Through anticipation-observation-reflection, you'll engage in meditation for relaxation and peace of mind as well as meditation for discovering and solving problems.

Through this process, you nurture self-awareness and creativity, you develop your own golf philosophy, and golf becomes more than a sport, growing into a lifetime path to self-mastery. And these experiences start manifesting their power in other areas of your life, too. There may be ways of doing the dishes, mopping the floor, washing the dog, and watering the flowers that are somehow different, somehow better. You can put more heart into such tasks, doing them with intention and devotion.

The brain is at the center of all life phenomena and human experience. Meditation in golf is a way of shining a bright light on your game by using consciousness, which is an operation of the brain. It's about looking dispassionately at your painful failures as well as the pleasant experiences of success, asking your own questions, and finding your own answers. In golf, as in all other experiences, to solve the problems you face, you ultimately have no choice but to rely on your own body and brain. You can get advice and help from experts, but that will mean nothing unless you experience the answers with your body and realize their truths with your brain. In golf, your greatest teachers are your body and brain, and meditation is a door to the wisdom they hold.

Don't Be Attached—Focus

We all know that we need to focus to be good at golf. However, sometimes when we think we're focusing, we're actually just getting attached to a particular outcome. Instead of focusing clearly on the here and now, attachment causes our minds to react to illusions of the past or future. Focus and attachment are similar in that they both involve concentrating awareness on something. The difference is that when you're focused, your consciousness is present and goal-oriented, but when you're attached, your consciousness is greed-oriented and located somewhere else.

When you focus, your emotions disappear. True focus leaves no room for attachment because you're putting all your awareness into the experience you're having here and now. But when you're attached to something, greedy emotions consume you. When things are going well, attachment stimulates excessive pride and arrogance, often causing you to lose focus. And when things go south, you can't help but react with frustration and anxiety. So, one way to distinguish between focus and attachment is to look at whether you are emotionally stable or not.

Your pre-shot routine should help you focus on the feeling of your swing with a stable, confident mind. Of course, you should clearly visualize your intended shot, but you must let go of the fear of messing up. Obsessing over not making a mistake, or being greedy about hitting the perfect shot, will make you impatient and anxious. Anxiety and impatience will cause you to lose the sense of your swing. Naturally, when this happens, your shot will not go where you intended.

By focusing without being attached, you can hit better shots. Because you are not attached to greed, you can relax after you hit the shot. And looking back without attachment over the experience of the shot you've just made lets you learn more. Attachment, on the other hand, leads to obsessing over missed shots, and it will keep you from focusing on your next shot.

Maintain Relaxed Concentration

There are expressions you frequently hear when you ask golfers who've played for more than a decade to describe the state of immersion they feel while playing. "I had no thoughts in my mind at all." "Time seemed to stand still." "It was like everything around me had stopped." "It was like I was the only one on the golf course, and I was completely unaware of the people around me."

All these comments refer to a meditative state in which relaxed concentration is maintained. The term "relaxed concentration" seems contradictory at first. Usually we're tense when focused, and our awareness wanders when we start to relax. To be successful in golf, however, you should be in a state of clarity with your tension relaxed and your awareness focused in the here and now. Relaxed concentration is a state in which you empty your mind to allow for free movement while you pay close attention to that movement.

Our attention spans are naturally limited. Just like you develop muscle pain and fatigue when using your muscles for a long time, your cranial nerves can be fatigued by maintaining focus for more than a certain period. So, we usually feel tense and tired if we concentrate for too long on a particular object or task. In contrast, meditation focuses on awareness without tension. That's why meditation is actually restful, relaxing your nerves instead of taxing them. Being in this state stabilizes your brain waves, heightening your sense of peace and fulfillment.

The words I've used to explain a state of immersion in golf are surprisingly similar to descriptions of energy meditation. When you feel energy, time flows slowly, space expands to infinity, and you feel at one with everything, as if the boundaries between you and your surroundings have disappeared. Feeling energy itself is already a meditation.

You can feel what relaxed concentration is through your energy sense. Depending on your mental focus, you'll be able to detect subtle changes in the density and direction of energy. Maintaining this feeling while playing golf will significantly improve your concentration and sense of being fully in the moment. Best of all, it can give you greater control over your body and mind.

Where Your Energy Goes, the Golf Ball Follows

There is a critical energy principle that you can apply to your golf: "Where the mind goes, energy follows."

If you've ever been in the zone, you've probably noticed that your mind had reached the state of relaxed concentration described in the previous pages. In golf, this is the optimal state of mind. Why? Most golfers know that having too many different thoughts while you swing is a recipe for disaster. For long-term consistency and success, being able to calm your mind and focus exclusively on the process of achieving your goal is priceless. When we're under pressure, the thoughts in our heads tend to multiply, scattering our focus.

The implication of this principle—where your mind goes, energy follows—is that when you have too many thoughts, not only is your focus scattered, but your energy is scattered.

Studying this principle as originally written in Korean brings more insight. In Korean, the principle is known as *shim ki hyeol jung*. This literally translates as "mind, energy, blood, matter." So the implication is that when your energy is scattered, your body tends to react with a similar "scatteredness." Then, when it comes time to swing the club, not only is your mind unfocused, but your body isn't primed to execute. In fact, your body is unconsciously taking cues from your mind and preparing to do a dozen things at once. In the case of those first-tee jitters, your body may be getting messages to run and hide, keep smiling, and get ready to throw up. With something as sensitive as a golf swing—where an adjustment of just a hundredth of an inch can make the difference between a birdie and a bogey, or worse—being able to focus your attention on the proper action is invaluable.

Recognizing that your mind affects your body will change the way you approach golf. At the very least, you'll realize the importance of the mental game. But when you fully apply this principle to your life, it will help you maximize the impact of everything you have ever practiced.

No matter how great your powers of concentration are, you can't maintain deep focus throughout the four or five hours it usually takes to complete a round of golf. You have to immerse yourself in the shot for 30 to 40 seconds, come out of it, and then instantly immerse yourself again when it's your turn. Even when joking and laughing with your companions, you should start your pre-shot routine and have a sense of instantaneous immersion when you get close to the ball. You need a sense of quickly returning to the here and now. You can only play golf in the here and now. If you let your mind wander to the shot you just made or the shot you'll make at the next hole even for an instant, you'll lose the shot you're making in the moment.

If you try the energy-sensing exercise introduced in the section on energy (page 70), you'll be able to get a real feel for the principle, "Where the mind goes, energy follows." You'll feel the energy in your hands when you focus your mind on your hands, and in your chest or abdomen when you focus your mind there. Like grass bending in the direction the wind blows, energy moves according to how you use your mind. This practice is extremely effective for developing concentration because your focus is immediately converted into changes in your body feeling. At first you feel the energy as you move your hands, but through steady practice you can maintain the feeling of energy even without moving your body.

All movements on the golf course—including swing, address, and putt—can be controlled much more sensitively if done while feeling the energy. You can reduce tension and anxiety on the course just by maintaining your energy sense. You can also put powerful energy into the golf ball by concentrating your mind.

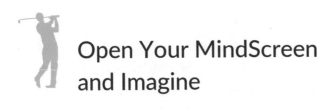

Open Your MindScreen and Imagine

One aspect of meditation that you're probably familiar with is visualization. This basically means using your imagination to picture things you want. It's powerful because imagining something activates many of the same responses in the brain as actually experiencing it.

For example, take a deep breath and imagine picking a bright yellow lemon from a tree. Feel the skin of the lemon in your hand. Now imagine taking a small, sharp knife and cutting the lemon in half. Inside, see the juicy lemon sections and a few seeds. Cut one piece in half again; lemon juice drips onto your fingers. Now bring that lemon quarter to your mouth and sink your teeth into it. Is your mouth watering? If so, you've got a good imagination and your body is responding. This same power can help on the golf course.

A U.S. Air Force colonel named George Hall was a prisoner of war in a POW camp in Vietnam for seven and a half years. A golf fanatic, he played 18 holes in his imagination every day. He imagined it so vividly that he was later able to control his swing and even the ball at will. He surprised many by shooting 76 in a golf tournament three weeks after returning home. "It was your first match, so you must have got lucky?" a reporter asked in an interview after the match. "Lucky?" Colonel Hall is said to have replied. "I haven't had a single three-putt in the last five years."

Many will be familiar with advice about visualizing your shot before you hit the ball. I like to quickly decide what shot I'm going to hit and then take a moment to visualize it as I stand over the ball. This is similar to the "See it" step from the "See it, Feel it, Trust it" method that some golf psychologists recommend, from the book *Seven Days in Utopia* by David L. Cook.

For many people, it's not the imagination or "seeing" part that's hard. It's that second step: feeling. Can you imagine a feeling? Can you transfer the image in your head to a feeling in your body? When I give lectures and seminars about health and wellness, I meet many people who complain about being unhappy. Some of them spend many minutes explaining the problems they're facing, what they've tried to do to fix them, and how they don't see a solution. After listening to a long list of issues, I ask them, "Can you smile now?" For some, the point is already made. If you want to be happy, don't over-complicate things. Yes, there are problems and challenges, but being happy is not about that.

For those who are really stuck, smiling becomes an actual exercise. I have them stretch their face muscles, making their smile bigger and bigger until they almost have tears in their eyes. Sometimes, I get everyone in the audience to practice moving their facial muscles. It can be quite a workout!

The disconnect between thinking and feeling is profound for far too many people. It can make us feel hopeless and apathetic when we intellectually understand something but aren't able to feel it. The same goes for golf. Too many of us suffer from being able to "see" the shot without being able to feel it. Then we try to "trust" it—but instead of trusting the feeling, we're trusting the imagination. As you know, you can't hit a real shot with nothing but your imagination. Feeling needs to be involved.

Hitting the ball without a clear feeling almost always results in a poor shot that doesn't match what we imagined. Then, we lose faith in our powers of visualization and employ all sorts of complicated mental gymnastics to make up for the fact that we now doubt ourselves.

See it, feel it, trust it. For 90 percent of people, I would say that the weak link is feeling. It's not a lack of imagination, and it's not even a limitation of the body; it's the lack of a bridge between them. That's why I keep emphasizing the importance of mind-body connection and introduce energy-sensing exercises throughout this book.

MindScreen meditation is a visualization exercise that helps to connect your energy sense (feeling) to your imagination. First, do the energy-sensing meditation introduced in the previous chapter. Repeatedly and slowly move your palms close together and then farther apart in front of your chest, feeling the energy. Try expanding the feeling of energy to your arm, and then to your whole body. Maintaining a sense of connection to the flow of energy, raise your hands to forehead height. Feel energy flowing into your brain and along your spine, spreading throughout your body. Sense the

The 100-Year Golfer

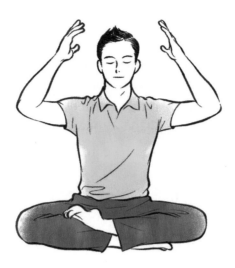

infinite space of consciousness unfolding in your brain. This is your MindScreen.

On your MindScreen, imagine the golf game you want to create in as much detail and as concretely as possible: the path of your swing, the vibrations transmitted to your hands and body at the moment of impact, the pleasant sound at impact, your companions shouting, "Good shot!", and the joy and happiness filling your heart. Mobilizing all your senses, imagine everything vividly, even your emotions.

As you imagine all these things, move your hands freely around your head, going with the feeling of energy. You can feel your golf game even more concretely through the sensations of energy. As your hands and energy move each other, you may at times even feel the distinction between them disappearing. The boundary fades so that you can't tell whether energy is moving your hands or your hands are moving energy. Everything is one within the harmonious flow of energy. When I introduced my own energy experience in the previous chapter, I described it as my body moving the instant I got some intention, as if my body was leading my intention. That's the feeling I'm talking about. In this dynamic give-and-take, the sensation of separation disappears, allowing you to be completely immersed in your imaginary golf game.

Once you're used to it, you can do MindScreen meditation without moving your hands or closing your eyes, while still maintaining a sense of energy. With regular practice, you can use it as one of your pre-shot routines on the golf course. At address, look at the ball while maintaining a sense of energy and quickly decide how you'll hit it. After picturing on your MindScreen the trajectory of the ball as it rises, falls, and rolls to a stop in the middle of the fairway, swing with confidence. Where the mind goes, energy follows. Where energy goes, the golf ball follows. Using your energy sense, bring your golf game to life—from your imagination to feeling to reality.

Rhythmic Movement
Becomes Meditation

As I've said before, meditation can be many different things. One practice I like to introduce to people is "dynamic meditation," basically meditation through movement. The simplest way to do it is through rhythmic body vibration, either standing, sitting, or lying down.

A standing body-bounce can induce meditative feelings in just a few seconds. Stand with your feet shoulder-width apart and bend your knees slightly. Relax your shoulders, take a deep breath, and begin to bounce gently up and down. Allow your shoulders and arms to bounce freely and heavily. Relax your back and leg muscles as much as you can without losing your balance. Let your neck and jaw muscles feel the vibration as well.

You can bounce quickly or slowly, whatever feels natural for your body. Exhale comfortably through your open mouth, as if you're breathing out tension and stress. Try it for a minute. Your brain may start buzzing with questions like, "What is this doing?" or "Do I look weird?" If that happens, exhale and keep going. Sticking to your plan no matter what

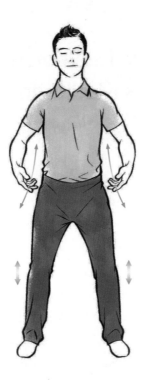

your thoughts and emotions do is part of what makes meditation effective. Do it now!

What do you notice afterward? Is there still a feeling of vibration in your body? Congratulations, you've already deepened your self-awareness. If you keep going, you'll start to notice your body temperature changing, your breathing getting deeper, your joints and muscles releasing stiffness, and your thoughts becoming simpler.

I like dynamic meditation because it may be easier than other types of meditation to apply to life situations, such as golf. Sitting and breathing quietly for 30 minutes is a wonderful way to meditate, and if you have the time and inclination, try it before playing a round of golf sometime. But for many of us, movement makes it easier to feel the impact of meditation.

Shake Your Head and Tap Your Belly

Another form of dynamic meditation using vibration is to tap your lower abdomen repeatedly and rhythmically with your fists while gently shaking your head from side to side. I call this Brain Wave Vibration because it quickly stabilizes brain waves.

When you're under stress, you start tensing up in your neck or, more precisely, in your first cervical vertebra, where the bones of your neck and skull meet. Lightly touch your index fingers to your ear canal openings and imagine a horizontal line connecting both fingers. Now imagine a line descending vertically from the crown of your head to the point where these two lines meet. The tension starts there.

Tension in the first cervical vertebra compresses the carotid artery in the neck, interfering with the supply of blood going into the brain and making the head heavy and hot. Unless relieved promptly, the tension that starts here travels down along the neck, making the entire neck stiff, and sinks into the shoulders and spine, making the whole upper body stiff. The most effective way to relieve this tension is to

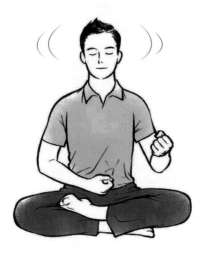

move the place where it began. The simplest and most natural way to release cervical tension is to shake your head gently from side to side like a baby. At the same time, make loose fists and gently tap your lower abdomen with the little-finger side of your fists. Exhale through your mouth at this time. Repeat for three to five minutes, then stop and breathe comfortably for one to two minutes, observing how your body feels.

Doing this releases tension in your neck, promoting the circulation of blood and energy flowing into your head and making your head feel refreshed. Rhythmically stimulating your lower abdomen generates heat, warming your belly. This creates the optimal state of energy balance—Water Up, Fire Down—with your head cool and belly warm, allowing you to naturally enter a state of relaxed concentration. It's even better if, after doing Brain Wave Vibration, you open your MindScreen and imagine your golf game. You can easily do both of these meditations in about 5 to 10 minutes.

Becoming a Single Golfer with Meditation

By Byeong-geun Min
48-year-old man, Seoul, South Korea, nine years of golf experience

I started playing golf nine years ago at the recommendation of my boss. At first, it felt awkward. I had pain in different places, including my lower back and wrists, and it was hard. I wondered why I had to play golf, but I had no choice since the sport was necessary for my business life.

At first, I was no different from any other ordinary golfer. I did repetitive practice at the practice range using the exact same movements, and when I got out on the course, I didn't know what I should do, which was embarrassing. There were even times when I felt stressed and wanted to give up.

After about three years, I wondered what would happen if I applied to golf the meditations I had learned at the Body & Brain Yoga center. On nights before I was supposed to play golf, prior to getting in bed, I would do about 30 minutes of toe tapping, focusing my awareness on the ends of my feet. I would do exercises to relax my whole body and strengthen my core and lower back. Later, I would close my eyes and do MindScreen meditation, breathing, and imagining swinging a golf club. I implanted in my brain a mindset that said, "I can move and control my body as I want." When I would do this before sleeping, I could get a good night's rest, and I was able to get good results on the course, playing with a very light body and mind. Meditation also helped a lot in the process of playing golf. Golf is a mental battle with yourself. You have to focus on yourself, not worry about whether you're doing well relative to your partners. You can't get good results if you golf with prejudice or a negative attitude.

Golf is a game that goes through a total of 18 holes, not ending because you do poorly on one. It's important to believe that you can do better on the next hole, even if you made mistakes on this one. Ruminating over your mistakes on the last hole and getting caught up in gradually more negative thinking often ruins the next hole. Through meditation, I used a positive mindset to erase my memory of the mistakes I'd made on the previous hole and, through a quick change of consciousness, to focus on the current hole.

When moving for my next shot, I would walk, step by step, over the grass while doing walking meditation, relaxing the tension in my body and controlling my breathing. When I would take a shot with the belief that I could be one with my golf club, I found that I could make an accurate impact, sending the ball where I wanted it to go.

Through meditation, I've gained the confidence that I can do anything. As a result, I've been able to become a single-digit handicapper and have even been lucky enough to make a hole-in-one. Lately, I've been teaching my wife and the people around me how to play golf using meditation. Now, through meditation, I've not only become a better golfer, but I've elevated the golf experience of my companions.

Create Your Own Swing with Qigong

My First and Last Golf School Experience

In the early days of my self-taught golf, I had this one worry: I wasn't getting any distance on my shots. Quite a few amateur female golfers drive the ball 220 yards, but my drives were only going between 165 and 185 yards.

An acquaintance who was playing golf with me, seeing me struggling with the driver, gave me a hint: "You're just hitting the ball hard, without rotating your body enough. With that kind of swing, your distance will never increase, even if you try your whole life. I think you should switch to a swing with a big arc."

At his urging, I enrolled at a golf academy, the first time I'd ever done such a thing. "If you go there, you can definitely learn how you should change your swing," he said. He'd boasted that 280 yards was an average drive for him, but the real reason he caught my attention was that the academy he suggested taught the secret of Greg Norman's swing. With Norman's prodigious length off the tee, his aggressive golf style, his blonde hair, and his Australian nationality, it's no wonder his nickname is the "Great White Shark."

It took me a whole day to travel from my home in Arizona to the academy in Florida. The program was mainly for people who wanted to become golf coaches, but because anyone could sign up, there were a lot of bogey players like me. During my week there, I learned the basics of the Greg Norman swing and various techniques, including how to hit a bunker shot and how to get a ball out of a divot.

Looking at my swing, the instructor pointed out that I should straighten my left arm. I was already working on the theory that I'd only be able to hit a long drive if I straightened my left arm to increase my swing arc and accelerate my head speed. It was more than a little difficult to execute this, though. When I'd straighten my arm, my posture would stiffen, and my golf club felt twice as heavy when I raised and lowered it to hit the ball. I'd swing with my arm straight, but far from sending the ball flying into the distance, my head speed would drop even more. Occasionally, though the ball might go some distance, its direction would be way off, leaving me flustered and embarrassed.

Even after returning from the program, I tried to straighten my arms as much as possible. But the more I did this, the less fun golf was. When I swung the way I was used to swinging, my ball would fly straight, if not far. When I'd try to straighten my arm, though, I produced all sorts of missed shots, duffing and topping the ball as if I were picking up a golf club for the first time. Eventually, I even began to lose my motivation to play. After a few months, I stopped trying to straighten my left arm and went back to my previous form.

Changing your swing is like major surgery. Even the pros are said to take one to two years to get their bodies used to a new driver swing. Continuing to study my swing, I later realized that trying to force my arm to straighten made my arms, shoulders, neck, and back tense, and tightening up my grip hurt my accuracy and head speed. The key was letting my arms hang without tension. Would I have been able to fix my swing had I realized the importance of relaxation then and practiced harder? I'm not sure. Now I swing with the muscles in my arms relaxed, but my left arm isn't completely straight. And I think that this posture fits my body better.

By the time I was close to 60, Sedona in Arizona had become my second home. The beauty of nature in Sedona has been a source of inspiration for me in my writing and business, as well as in golf. In fact, this was where golf changed for me, from being just a hobby to being a serious means of brain training and spiritual practice. It was about this time that I once again made up my mind to improve my swing form, and I started putting more time and energy into it.

As I began the project of creating Earth Village, an environmentally friendly lifestyle education facility in New Zealand, I started going between South Korea, New Zealand, and Sedona several times a year. During this time, mainly in New Zealand and Sedona, I got my body used to a new swing, practicing with a larger axis of rotation in my trunk that allowed me to drive the ball farther.

Swing without a Golf Ball or Club

It is no exaggeration to say that I've experienced all the trial-and-error that you'd expect a self-taught golfer to go through. In particular, I started with no understanding of swing path, so at first, I focused on swinging my golf club to hit the ball as hard as I could. For a long time, I golfed by striking with the power of my arms, without using my whole body. My ineffective swing mechanics became a habit, which was hard to change. Only after I'd been playing golf for 20 years did I find a more effective swing rhythm, one that's right for my body and allows me to continuously improve my game.

The key to the golf swing is creating a good arc and rhythm, not just hitting the ball. If you develop your swing path and tempo, the ball will go soaring even if you tell it not to. Anyone who hits the ball solidly has their consistent swing path and rhythm to thank for it. If you lose your rhythm or deviate from your natural swing path, greedy for distance, the golf ball will end up going to all the wrong places. You must trust your repeatable swing path and rhythm instead of being swept away by ever-changing thoughts and emotions.

How can you develop a good golf swing and find a swing rhythm that's natural for you? Reflecting on my own trial and error with these questions in mind, I devised Golf Meridian Exercise and Golf Qigong. These exercises can be done using only your body. How often do you practice your golf swing without even using a club? Many people take practice swings without a golf ball, but to practice without a club in your hands may seem a bit strange. If you observe yourself closely, however, you'll notice that concentrating too much on the ball creates anxiety and tension. And when you grasp your golf club, you may be more concerned with swinging the club than with moving your body. That's why I'm advising you to spend some time concentrating fully on the movement of your body as you swing, without using a golf ball or club.

For beginners, practicing the basic movements of the swing with Golf Meridian Exercise will help you create a swing that is more relaxed and balanced. If you're a golfer who has already mastered the basics of the golf swing, Golf Qigong will help you find a swing that's powerful but natural and smooth, flowing like water, and a golf rhythm that's right for your body.

Relax and Balance Your Body with Golf Meridian Exercise

"Relaxing," it is commonly said among South Korean golfers, "takes three years." Many golfers, though, have trouble truly relaxing even after 10 or 20 years. Unless your body relaxes, the parts you *should* move get all mixed up with those you *shouldn't*. Your center of gravity is shaken, and your swing arc and rhythm are disturbed, making it impossible to impact the ball properly.

Golf Meridian Exercise helps you develop a sense of how to relax your body. The movements push and pull the muscles and tendons, eliminating tension and relaxing the body. They also push and pull the meridians of the body, the pathways through which energy flows, so that energy can move unimpeded through them for more profound relaxation. The principles involved aren't all that different from golf itself, in which a swing follows a semi-circle, making an arc by pushing for half the circle and then pulling for the other.

There's something I often hear non-golfers say: "Is golf even exercise? The whole thing is riding a cart, walking for a little bit, then occasionally hitting a ball. Do you even break a sweat?" We golfers chuckle when we hear things like that. Playing 18 holes in four or five hours takes a lot of high-intensity energy, mentally and physically. What's more, amateurs go out on the course and hit around 80 to 110 balls (with the goal of reducing that number). And out of sight, they practice a lot just to play a single round of golf. In fact, they end up exercising a lot more while practicing than while playing on the course.

People who frequent the golf course and practice range should pay special attention to correcting the disordered balance of their bodies. Golf involves rotating the body only to one side, which can easily injure the neck, lower back, and hip joints. If you continue swinging only to one side when you practice, your body's imbalance inevitably gets worse. I've even known someone who cracked a rib from rotating his torso too much while practicing enthusiastically.

I created Golf Meridian Exercise 15 years ago to help people golf in a way that's a little healthier, more comfortable, and more enjoyable, and I've upgraded it several times since then. The program is made up of 11 exercises: a warmup, nine main exercises, and a cooldown activity. The focus is on learning the torso rotation, hip turn, and arm, shoulder, and leg movements used in the golf swing while simultaneously relaxing muscles and joints and developing a sense of centering the body. Also, exercising in the opposite direction helps prevent injury and restore the body's balance. Don't pick up your golf club at the driving range until you have sufficiently warmed up with Golf Meridian Exercise!

The 100-Year Golfer

It's hard to fully understand the exercise movements from text and pictures alone, but you can learn the practice by watching videos on the Ilchi Brain Golf channel on YouTube. The following Golf Meridian Exercises will be shown as a sequence in one video. Use the QR code on page 166 to access the YouTube video.

Repeat each of the movements 30 to 50 times until you're warm and sweating. For the exercises that involve deep breathing, do 5 to 10 repetitions. What's important is producing a satisfactory change in your body, not how many repetitions you do. The trick is to repeat the motions until you feel sufficiently warmed up and your movements feel natural. These are good warmup exercises to do when standing on the first tee box at the golf course as well as at the practice range.

Keep these four rules in mind as you do all the exercises:

1. Move your weight into the soles of your feet, emptying your head and feeling balanced in your center.

2. Focus on your body, observing the movements of your muscles and joints, looking for any stiffness or discomfort, and feeling the energy.

3. Raise your arms with power generated from the soles of your feet and then lower your arms, simply using gravity to let them drop.

4. Move your body in both directions so that it doesn't develop imbalance on one side.

Warmup: Breath Control

Bring your feet together and balance yourself, letting your weight settle into your feet. Inhale, raising your arms up above your head, and then exhale, pointing your palms down and lowering your hands toward your legs. Repeat three to five times, moving as if you are sweeping the front of your body with energy.

This movement gently loosens your arms, shoulders, and spine, helping you focus on your body through breathing. As you sweep the front of your body with your hands, your awareness naturally turns inward toward your center. This helps you relax and improves your body awareness.

Golf Meridian Exercises
YouTube Video

1. Core Twists

Stand comfortably with your feet shoulder-width apart. Bend your knees about five degrees and let your weight sink into your feet. Stand so you have the feeling that you're grasping the ground with your feet. Without moving your head or feet, lightly twist your hips left and right, feeling your core moving. Let your arms follow along, wrapping around your body naturally. Fix your gaze on a point to the front and 45 degrees downward. Repeat this movement 30 to 50 times.

You've probably already done this unconsciously on the golf course to relieve a stiff back. This movement twists your body gently to warm up your spine and core. It's important to firmly fix your feet on the ground and not twist your torso too far. Relax your upper body and feel the power of your core. This movement helps warm up your important core muscles and develop your balance and flexibility.

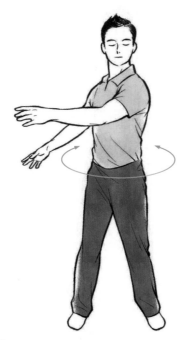

2. Vertical Arm Swings

Stand comfortably with your feet shoulder-width apart. Bend your knees about 5 to 15 degrees and keep the soles of your feet firmly stuck to the floor. Alternately move your arms in front of you up and down, feeling the force pushing them up from the soles of your feet and then letting gravity take over when you drop them. Do 30 to 50 repetitions.

A golf swing harmoniously connects the movements of different parts of your body. This movement relaxes your arms, shoulders, and upper back by alternately shaking your arms up and down. It also helps release muscle tension from your shoulders to your fingertips and improves your control and the sensitivity of your hands.

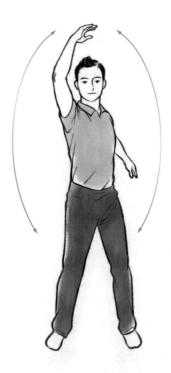

3. Horizontal Arm Swings

Stand comfortably with your feet shoulder-width apart. Bend your knees about five degrees and let your weight sink into your feet. Holding your arms in front of you about 45 degrees, swing them to the left and the right. Without moving your head or feet, fix your gaze on a point to the front and 45 degrees downward. When you swing your arms, your torso and spine will naturally follow along. Do 30 to 50 repetitions.

This exercise helps with smooth rotational movements of the shoulders, arms, chest, and back. Let your arms move naturally around your body without over-twisting your torso or over-swinging your arms. Fix your feet firmly to the floor to keep your balance.

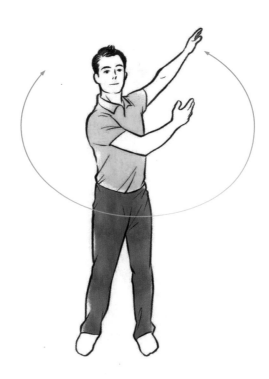

4. Full-Body Twists

Standing with your feet shoulder-width apart, raise your arms about 45 degrees in front of you, shift your weight to one foot, and bend the opposite knee, rotating it inward. Turn your bent knee until it lightly touches the opposite leg, and lift your heel off the ground as in a golf swing. Fix your gaze to the front and 45 degrees downward, and let your upper body follow the twisting of your lower body, feeling your arms rising higher than your shoulders and your torso and spine rotating. Shift your weight and swing to the other side. Focus on balance, rhythm, and relaxation. Do 30 to 50 repetitions.

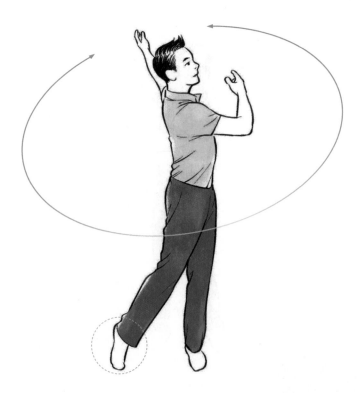

5. Bent-Over Shake

This movement may seem a little odd, but it helps strengthen and stretch the core muscles that you need for your golf swing. Spread your feet shoulder-width apart and clasp your hands together in front of you. Bend forward from the waist about 90 degrees, extending your arms in front of you while keeping your knees slightly bent. Raising your head, look to the front while keeping your spine relaxed. In this position, flex your lower abdomen and move your hips from side to side in a wavelike motion. Move your buttocks and arms, too. Focus on maintaining the feel of your core and your balance. Do about 30 repetitions.

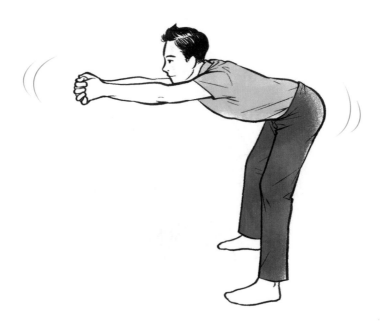

6. Energy Grounding

If you've ever seen a tai chi demonstration, this posture will be familiar to you. The movement of the arms is prominent, but the lower body is the key.

Stand comfortably with your feet shoulder-width apart, your knees slightly bent, and your tailbone tucked in. Feel your core muscles tensing slightly. Inhale, slowly raising your arms in front of you until they reach high above your head, imagining them floating above the clouds. Hold your breath a little and feel your chest expanding. Exhale, slowly lowering your arms as if moving them in water. (Those who have high blood pressure should raise their arms only to eye level and take care to breathe comfortably without holding their breath.) Do three to five repetitions.

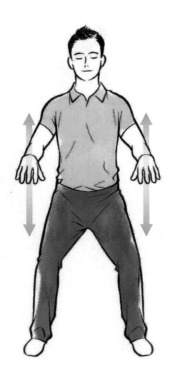

The 100-Year Golfer

7. Tiger Claw Posture

Stand with your feet together and your knees slightly bent, about five degrees. Inhale and curl your toes, grasping the ground with your feet. At the same time, flex your fingers and wrists to make your palms into "tiger claws" and slowly raise both arms to belly-button height. Now hold your breath for a moment, feeling power and energy entering your feet, fingers, and wrists. While exhaling, relax your wrists, fingers, and toes as your arms drop.

Repeat three to five times. This movement will help develop strength and flexibility in the feet and hands, particularly in the wrists.

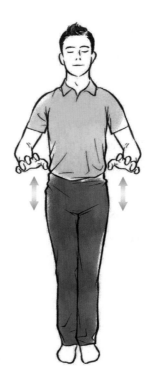

8. Chest-Spine Stretching

In traditional Korean medicine, the Conception Vessel (a meridian flowing along the midline of the front of the body) and the Governor Vessel (a meridian flowing along the midline of the back of the body) are very important. The Water Up, Fire Down principle introduced in the section on energy is closely related to the energy cycle of these two meridians. A body with opened Conception and Governor meridians develops vitality and achieves balance and harmony. The following movements open these two meridians, making your body more relaxed, awake, and balanced.

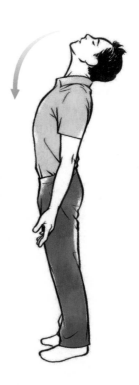

Stand with your feet spread shoulder-width apart. Relax your shoulders comfortably and inhale, tilting your neck slowly backward as if you're trying to touch the back of your head to your upper back. Now exhale, bending your neck and upper body forward as if you're trying to touch your chin to your chest.

Repeat these motions three to five times. You may lose your balance or feel dizzy, so work with the weight of your body sinking into your feet and the soles of your feet firmly planted on the ground.

The 100-Year Golfer

9. Twisting Horse Stance

For these modified qigong movements, stand with your feet shoulder-width apart and your knees bent about 15 degrees. Feel the stability of your weight sinking into your feet and your feet gripping the ground. With your tailbone curled in and your core muscles flexed, inhale and raise your hands to chest height, bending your wrists back. Gently tighten your lower abdomen, hold your breath, and twist your upper body to one side as far as you can. Keep your hips and knees bent, without moving your legs. Then exhale, turning your upper body back to the front and slowly lowering your hands. Now do the same thing in the opposite direction.

Repeat these motions three to five times. You can do this exercise quickly and rhythmically, but it's crucial to maintain balance and control and to keep your core muscles gently flexed.

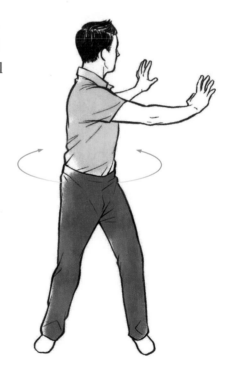

Cooldown: Energy Control

Spread your feet shoulder-width apart and bring your hands together in front of your chest. Now inhale, raise your hands with palms together, and extend your arms above your head. Bending your elbows, lower your hands behind your neck and extend your arms outward, pressing your palms to the left and right; hold your breath for a moment. Then exhale, bringing your feet together and putting your palms on your lower back. Bend your upper body forward, sweeping your palms downward from your lower back to the backs of your legs and heels. Stand up slowly, spread your feet shoulder-width apart again, and repeat the exercise three to five times.

Find Your Swing Rhythm with Golf Qigong

You've probably heard this saying a lot: "Swing within your limits." The best golfers in the world have great bodies and a great sense of movement, but they also have their own limitations in strength, flexibility, and sense of coordination. And what about us amateurs? How can we maximize our abilities within our limits to make the most efficient swing? Golf Qigong was developed as an answer to this question. Qi refers to energy, the feeling and flow of vital life force. Gong refers to form, postures, and movements that maintain and even amplify the energy.

To hit within your limits means to swing naturally. Of course, to swing with a golf club you must use force. The question is how you can use only the necessary amount of power. It takes constant practice to know how much force your swing requires. If you use more power than you need for your swing, the swing arc loses its naturalness, and the ball doesn't travel the way you want it to.

The swing that feels natural will differ for each golfer, depending on that individual's physique, physical condition, and golf experience. Unable to make a full swing, 102-year-old Jongjin Lee could only raise and lower his club. Even so, he consistently hit 150 yards and bogeyed several holes. He had his own balanced swing rhythm.

Learning to maximize your ability within your limits is one of the most important and productive things to focus on. Best of all, anybody can benefit from this practice, regardless of age, condition, or background.

"Sure," you might say, "I understand that playing within my limits would be good, but how do I actually practice that?" I'd like to suggest that qigong is one of the best ways to develop all the qualities you'll need to play within your limits. Through qigong, you can maximize your strength and flexibility while maintaining balance and relaxation.

Swing Qigong

We all want to hit the driver farther, straighter, and more consistently. I want to emphasize three things as the most important qualities needed to achieve this: balance, comfort, and repeatability.

Your driver swing needs to match what your body and mind can do every time you are on the tee. When you swing your driver, each part of the swing must stay under control and in balance. Get rid of all your thoughts of looking like a pro and crushing it 300 yards, even if that's something you can do. Instead, focus on staying under control, being in the flow, and exerting less than 70 percent of your maximum effort.

To practice Swing Qigong, you're going to start by setting aside your club. That's right, this swing practice is just you using your body. If you want to get a good sense of your limits, you have to start with just your body, nothing more.

Step One. The first step involves strengthening all the basic elements of the swing, from the ground up. Assume a comfortable stance, bending your knees and leaning your upper body forward. Let your arms hang comfortably from your shoulders. Practice rotating backward and forward from your shoulders, letting your elbows stay close to your rib cage. Make sure your balance isn't shifting to your toes or heels; keep it centered.

You will notice your weight shifting more to your back leg as you turn to the right (for a right-handed golfer) and more into your front leg as you turn to the left. Feel rooted to the ground through your feet, keeping your spine relaxed and stable. Like a tree with a strong trunk and roots that extend deep into the ground, feel the power to initiate your swing coming from your lower body, and maintain that feeling throughout this practice.

Step Two. Now it's time to craft your swing. This is where your own unique physical characteristics will come into play.

Start with the same balanced setup as in Step One. Turn into your backswing, maintaining the strength and balance in your core. Find how far you can turn without losing this sense of balance and centeredness—it may be less than you expect. Respect this limit. Even though you might be used to making a more complete turn when swinging your driver, you're likely losing balance, power, and precision by allowing momentum to carry you beyond your natural limit.

Go slowly as you start your downswing. This is important. Swing Qigong works by filling in the gaps of strength and awareness in your swing. By going slowly, you'll force yourself to find the connection between the different positions in your swing.

I'm not going to try to direct you on what positions to hit, what angles to maintain, and so on. You likely have plenty of knowledge about that already. I'm simply going to emphasize these two things: go slowly and stay in balance.

If you can, practice in front of a mirror. How does your body feel as you slowly move from one position to the next? You should be very comfortable throughout this process. If you find yourself in a position where your body is straining or off-balance, then you have a choice to make. Either find a more natural, less taxing posture—even if it doesn't look like the pros on TV—or begin increasing your strength and flexibility through weeks or months of exercise.

I recommend that you never feel like you're using more than 70 percent of your maximum possible effort. One way to check this is by noticing whether you can hold still in each posture for a full minute, breathing comfortably. If not, those positions are probably too taxing for you.

Step Three. Once you've found the postures that work for your body at each position, it's time to practice flowing between them. This is where we start to practice real qigong. To develop your sense of energy, I recommend that you try the energy-sensing exercise introduced in the energy section.

The 100-Year Golfer

It can help awaken your body awareness, develop your feel and touch around the greens, and enable you to focus your mind. This will be increasingly important as we talk about chipping and putting.

As you move through the natural postures you've identified as healthy for your body, concentrate on your hands. Focus on the feeling of energy in your hands. This could be warmth, pulsation, or even pressure or a magnetic sensation. Maintain your awareness of that feeling through your swing. Feel how the sensation changes in each position during your swing.

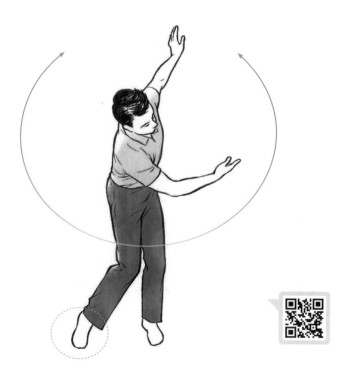

Imagine the moment of impact: all your body's energy coursing into your hands, through the club, and into the ball. Visualize and feel this process as you move slowly through your swing. Staying relaxed and balanced, you'll notice the feeling of power in your hands increasing. If you strain your body or lose your balance, however, you'll unconsciously be pulling energy away from your hands as you try to recover.

Have fun with this process! Your movements can become like a dance in which you push and pull energy with your hands. You can strengthen and stretch your body through this qigong movement, all the while maintaining your balance and centeredness. Practice for 5, 10, or even 20 minutes to find your natural flow. You'll build power, precision, and overall health. You may even find this movement meditative and relaxing.

Step Four. Finally, you're ready to grab your driver! But don't let everything you've worked on disappear. Imagine that the driver is simply an extension of your hands. Go slowly through each position. Feel the energy flowing from your feet to your core, through your spine to your shoulders and arms. Feel powerful energy channeled to your hands and through the club into the ball.

I guarantee that even if you feel like you're not swinging as hard as before, you're going to hit the ball more solidly, and probably straighter and farther, than you ever have. And you'll feel good doing it!

Chipping Qigong

According to Sam Snead, who—along with Tiger Woods—holds the PGA Tour record for most wins (82), "You can't do proper body rotation unless your muscles allow it. Even so, if you can chip and putt well, you can still get a good score." Those are enticing words for middle-aged-and-older golfers who feel their strength isn't what it used to be.

Chipping the ball obviously requires a simpler motion than a full golf swing, and yet for many people it can be even more challenging. What can qigong do to help you improve? For something so simple, the key is not to overthink it. Chipping Qigong is all about stability and feel. You want to have a consistent motion that your body can trust.

Chipping Qigong will help you develop two aspects of your chipping. First, you'll work on creating a stable and repeatable body motion that puts your hands in a comfortable position to chip the ball. Then you'll work on something that I call "hand intelligence," a technique for developing more strength, sensitivity, and awareness in your hands.

Step One. Start with whatever stance is comfortable for you. Set aside your club and get into position, bending your knees and leaning forward from the waist. Now shift your weight into your forward leg (the left leg, for a right-handed player). You may want to exaggerate your weight shift to further develop your balance.

Lean forward and let your arms hang comfortably from your shoulders. Let your palms face each other, keeping about 3 or 4 inches between them. This will be important when you move on to the next step.

Now practice moving your upper body "triangle." The goal here is to minimize the amount of sway, both side to side and up and down, in your chipping motion. Practice turning from your waist, moving slowly back and forth through the chipping motion so that your arms don't *swing* but just turn with your body. You can also apply whatever chipping tips and techniques work for you.

Step Two. Once your motion feels stable and consistent, begin to focus on your hands. You want your hands to remain as comfortable as possible throughout the motion. You should be able to sense your palms and the space between them as you move. This doesn't mean that your hands should be limp—keep your fingers "alive" without straining. Tightening your shoulders or elbows too much will reduce the feeling in your hands. Your goal is to make this motion as consistent and balanced as possible, letting you relax and put your hands in the best possible position.

Golf, like many sports, relies heavily on the use of the hands; it requires *hand intelligence*. Our hands tend to be one of the body's most sensitive areas, with an extraordinary number of nerve endings. The sensitivity, as well as strength, of your hands can be enhanced with meditations such as the energy-sensing exercise introduced in the energy section. When you connect this sensitivity with the power of your imagination, you develop the feel that is incredibly important in golf, especially in chipping and putting. Bringing your awareness to your hands as you do Chipping Qigong, linking body and mind, also serves as a form of meditation itself.

Step Three. Now that you've practiced making your chipping motion simple and stable and developed the awareness in your hands, let's put the two together. Take your stance and let your arms hang comfortably from your shoulders. Once you feel the sensation between your palms while in your golf stance, begin to move your hands gently farther apart and then closer together. Keep your shoulders relaxed and breathe comfortably. Begin moving through your chipping motion, keeping some space between your palms. Try to maintain the feeling between your palms throughout the chipping motion. Practice this as much as you can.

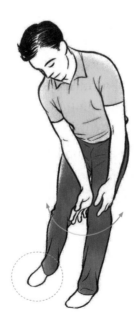

Step Four. Now it's time to transfer your awareness from your hands to the club. This may be a revelatory experience for you, especially if you're new to sensing energy.

Nearly every golf instructor emphasizes the importance of the grip. Why is this? It's because the grip is the foundation of how awareness is transferred from the body into the club. Is there a perfect grip? Like most things in life, probably not. But it's worth studying the fundamentals of a good grip as laid out by golfing professionals.

I'd like you to work on developing awareness through your grip. A grip that allows you the same sensitivity you had while practicing the energy sensing meditation will be better than a grip that distracts or dulls your awareness. The intelligence of your hands must be trusted if you're to hit or chip the golf ball the way you intend to.

Practice chipping the ball with the same awareness as you had when doing Chipping Qigong without your club, feeling the weight, pressure, and even the magnetic sensations in your hands and club. For most people, the error will be gripping the club too tightly, dulling awareness.

Now practice, practice, practice—but always with awareness. Aim to stay in the zone throughout your practice session and on the course, and your powers of relaxed concentration will increase. Not only will this help you improve your chipping, but it will obviously be useful in your overall game.

Putting Qigong

Putting is the most important shot in a golf game in terms of frequency. Statistics show that putting accounts for about 43 percent of all strokes, regardless of skill. You should invest at least a third of your practice time in putting, since it has a lot of impact on the game.

Of all the aspects of golf that test mind and body, putting is certainly one extreme. Precise feel, control, and imagination are essential if you want to be a good putter, and the hand intelligence that I previously described is more important than anything else. I believe that anyone, regardless of their ability level, can become an above-average putter simply by working on Putting Qigong.

Step One. Putting Qigong, like Swing Qigong and Chipping Qigong, starts with the stance. For Putting Qigong, it's even more important that your stance is perfectly balanced and relaxed. Your goal should be to put your hands in the most natural position throughout your putting stroke, thereby maximizing your feel and control.

Start again by taking your stance without your putter and allowing your arms to hang comfortably from your shoulders. Check that your back isn't straining and that your weight is centered in the soles of your feet.

Step Two. Now focus on your palms, feeling the space between them. Make subtle adjustments to your posture until you feel the magnetic sensation between your hands most strongly. This may mean adjusting your spine angle, bending your knees more or less, or moving your arms a degree closer to or farther from your body. No two players will be exactly the same, even though the general foundation of putting is similar. Now, with strong awareness of your hands, practice making a controlled turn with your shoulders and arms.

Step Three. When you're ready, add the putter. As you hold it, try to recapture the same awareness that you had when you were using just your hands. Feel the extra weight of the putter, but rather than tensing your arms to swing it, relax and use your core and lower body more than when you were moving only your arms. In this way, you can maintain feel and balance.

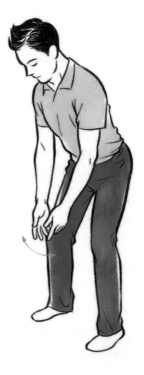

The 100-Year Golfer

Golf, a Game That's All Your Own

Ultimately, qigong is about finding your own natural flow and rhythm. When done well, qigong feels like a dance full of power, balance, and flowing movements, or like a song with perfect harmony. A golf swing is like singing, dancing, or playing an instrument. Have you ever been touched by the beauty and emotion in a song you were singing? Even if you can't sing very well, the sound can be beautiful if the rhythm is alive, fits your breathing, and is rich in emotion.

The same goes for your golf swing. When we swing in the way that's most natural to us, we feel beauty in ourselves. Our body becomes an instrument for expressing ourselves. In golf, that instrument expresses its rhythm through the golf club. Practicing Golf Qigong, you'll find that your swing is not merely an action for hitting a ball. A swing is a dance, a qigong, a song, and an expression of your life.

When we watch the world's very best players, we often marvel at the beauty and control in their games. There's no substitute for the hours and hours of practice that professionals spend honing their skills, but everyone can tap into their own natural flow through qigong. Rather than being machines making the same perfectly mechanical swing each time, we can aspire to be artists expressing our inner power and creativity in each moment. If you focus on this, even though you may not play perfect golf, you'll play golf that is perfectly your own.

Learning New Techniques Easily Thanks to Golf Qigong

By David Driscoll
40-year-old man, Phoenix, USA, six years of golf experience

I n high school, I was a baseball and soccer player. I first tried golf on a whim one summer under the guidance of my neighbor. My only recollection from those few summer rounds is of topping drives off the first tee and utilizing my baseball swing as best I could, spraying the ball wildly across the course.

In my 30s, I once again discovered golf. I literally discovered it in the form of a set of used golf clubs on the side of the road. I parked my car one morning and saw the clubs sitting near the curb. When I returned in the afternoon they were still there, and I took it as a sign that someone had finally quit the game or simply couldn't pack them at the end of their lease.

I took my newfound clubs to a local driving range, purchased a bucket of golf balls, and proceeded to blister my hands over the next hour. I managed to connect solidly on about one out of every 10 shots, and that was enough. After that, I was hooked.

Like many amateur golfers, a lot of my learning was through YouTube videos, books, and watching other golfers on the course. I had the privilege to learn the principles and methods of Ilchi Brain Golf directly from Ilchi Lee, and the experience supercharged my ability to integrate new information into my golf practice. One of the ways that I integrate new techniques is through Golf Qigong.

If you're already familiar with qigong, you'll know it's a form of meditative or healing martial arts. It combines balance, strength, and coordination exercises through a series of postures and flowing movements. For me, Golf Qigong has become a go-to method of turning new ideas into tangible feelings and actions.

It doesn't take much time to understand new techniques. But incorporating them into the golf swing takes significant practice and repetition, and that's where Golf Qigong helps.

Let's say I'm watching a video about getting my weight onto my lead leg. When I go to practice with the club, it will be difficult to avoid slipping into old habits. Through Golf Qigong, I can get out of my head and create a new feeling. Golf Qigong is slow enough that I can maintain balance and connection without being "mechanical." I still feel how the swing will flow, where the power and energy are concentrated, and how I'll be able to incorporate the new feeling into my full-speed swing.

Bring Self-Care
and Self-Healing
to Your Golf

Be Sure to Recharge after Practice

As we get older, we can remember the feeling of playing our best game when we were younger. Our brains haven't forgotten how to hit a drive long and straight or how to line up a putt, but often our bodies don't respond the way they used to. On the right day, though, when we're feeling strong and flexible, we can recapture the natural ability that we once enjoyed and that our brains still expect.

Interestingly, this experience isn't limited to older athletes. Professional athletes of all ages have to deal with the effects of continuous exertion and physical stress. In highly competitive, physically demanding sports, such as boxing, football, or rugby, competitors will rarely be fully healthy during a season. Bumps, bruises, and worse can take a toll, not only on physical strength, but also on the basic ability of the body and brain to communicate, which affects balance, coordination, and even concentration.

Even gentler, less physically taxing sports—like golf—involve a certain amount of physical exertion, especially in the repetition of specific movements. Over time, accumulated stress can cause physical weakness, tension, and a loss of coordination. As we get older, this will only intensify.

I'd like to suggest how to look at your long-term progress and health in golf and in daily life, especially as you grow older. If you are serious about playing golf for a lifetime, then put 50 percent of your effort into self-healing and recovery.

You've no doubt heard of "rest and recovery." These days, professional athletes regularly practice "load management" to reduce the likelihood of injuries. But I want to use the term "self-healing" because, to me, the proactive nature of taking care of your body isn't captured by "rest and recovery." To maximize your self-healing ability, you must work actively to release tension from your body and get the energy flowing.

After a round of golf, you might notice that your body feels tight. Perhaps your back is stiff or sensitive. If you walked the course, maybe your legs are sore, or your hips feel tight. Or maybe your wrists or knees ache. But if you want to improve your game, it's essential to get back to practicing or playing as soon as you can. How can you get your body ready to play more quickly? You need to practice self-healing.

The Day I Hit 12 Jumbo Boxes of Golf Balls

There have been times when I've practiced golf so hard that I stupidly overdid it. In my mid-40s, when there were around 50 Body & Brain Yoga centers in South Korea, I moved to the United States to fulfill my dream of teaching the world the mind-body training and meditation methods that I'd developed. Putting down roots in a strange land with an unfamiliar culture and language wasn't easy. Rushing here, running there, I found myself in an endless cycle of trial-and-error.

One of the members at a Body & Brain Yoga center in New Jersey just happened to be running a golf range at the time. Hearing that I played golf, he arranged for me to come and practice whenever I wanted. I went to his driving range whenever I was frustrated and didn't see a way ahead. It's probably accurate to say that I went more to cool off my overwhelmed, overheated brain than to practice golf.

I've stressed in this book that you should practice with your mind and body connected, but I was far from setting such an example back then. My body was wielding a golf club, but my head was a jumble of thoughts about my predicament at the time: "What should I do to spread Brain Education in America?" I hit a lot of golf balls in a short time, enough to shock the golfers in the next box over. There was even a day when I practiced from morning to evening, hitting 12 jumbo boxes containing 100 golf balls each. I walloped them, leaving my palms swollen and blistered. My left shoulder throbbed, my lower back ached, and my knees hurt. I even developed a mild case of tennis elbow.

On nights after such practices, I'd lie in bed trying to sleep, my body weary, when I'd find myself doing exercises. I'd extend my arms and legs, stretch my whole body, and shake and pat my body all over. I'd also lift my arms and legs, gathering energy in the Sleeping Tiger pose described in the breathing section. Rather than feeling like exercise, such movements were physiological phenomena arising automatically from my body to relieve fatigue, like yawning when you're sleepy. My body made me move like that to heal itself.

The throbbing pain subsided greatly after that, and my body became lighter, allowing me to sleep well. I was able to get up much more quickly in the morning. Now those natural healing movements created by my body have become one of my golf routines for quickly recovering and recharging my energy after a round or practice. And each time, I find myself saying, "Oh, that feels so good!" and feeling my body fill up with energy like a battery that's recharging.

I'm going to introduce a simple routine that I've found helpful in activating my body's self-healing ability. If you practice this routine after a day of golf, I believe you'll feel more refreshed and relaxed, and your body will recover much more quickly than it would otherwise.

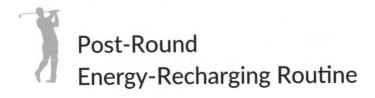

Post-Round
Energy-Recharging Routine

After practice or rounds of golf, this relaxation and energy-recharging routine will relieve tension in your tired body and mind, and calm parts of the body that have moved excessively.

Toe Tapping. Start by lying on your back on a yoga mat or other soft, but firm surface—this won't work well on your bed, for example. Stretch out your legs with your ankles together, and shake your feet back and forth like windshield wipers, letting your toes tap together. You should notice your leg muscles getting a little tired. Keep breathing comfortably, relaxing your shoulders. After one to two minutes, stop and breathe for 30 seconds, being aware of the sensations you feel in your legs. You may have a sense of continuing vibration or heaviness.

Knee Bouncing. Next, lift your knees up slightly, and then gently drop them down onto the mat. Feel the backs of your legs being stimulated, from heels to hips. Keep bouncing your knees for about 30 seconds. Start gently. This shouldn't be painful for your knee joints; if it is, skip ahead to the next movement. After 30 seconds of knee-bouncing, stop and feel the residual vibration in your leg muscles.

Hip Bouncing. Still lying on your back, bend your knees and place your feet flat on the floor. Starting gently, lift and drop your pelvis. You'll be simulating the sacrum or back of the pelvis. This can help release tension in the spine and hips. Breathe comfortably. After 30 seconds, stop and observe what you are feeling.

Back Bouncing. This final technique may not be possible for everyone, but give it a try. Press your elbows into the ground next to you and arch your spine up off the floor. Press the back of your head into the ground as you lift up your middle back and shoulder blades, then gently drop your spine. Repeat. It should feel like someone is tapping your back during a massage. Breathe out gently each time you drop your spine. Try to find a rhythm, and continue to do back bouncing for 20 seconds. Afterward, breathe deeply and feel the sensations in your rib cage and back muscles.

Repeat these four techniques until your body and mind feel more relaxed. In between, try a few simple stretching exercises such as hugging your knees to your chest, gently twisting one leg across your body, or stretching both arms over your head. You can also add in other stretches along with some core-strengthening and breathing exercises.

Above all, if you want to prepare your body for proper rest and recovery, you need to *move*. The repetitive motions of the golf swing will cause tension to accumulate in specific areas, and it's hard to release that tension if you don't move.

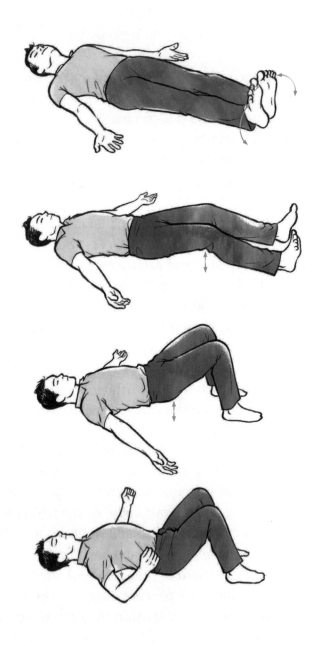

The 100-Year Golfer

Let me explain more about how the routine I've just outlined can help you. First, it will feel great to get off your feet and stretch out on your back. The toe tapping exercise helps activate circulation in your lower body, releases tension from your lower back, and deepens your breathing. You might be surprised at how challenging it can be, but don't give up. It will help you release pain and tension in your legs and back.

Knee bouncing is another great way to release tension in your leg muscles and get energy flowing. It can also help to realign your posture by stimulating both sides evenly. Hip bouncing is the same: great stimulation for a part of the body that can be difficult to stretch, strengthen, and relax. Relaxing and rebalancing your hip joints is one of the best ways to help your spine recover a healthy posture. Finally, back bouncing can help you release tension from your spine, neck, and shoulders, deepen your breathing, and calm your mind in case your round of golf left you slightly upset.

Golf relies on a subtle awareness of body movement, position, balance, and speed. Even the smallest amount of tension can interrupt the flow of information between your brain and body. Most of the time, we don't notice this accumulation of tension until it has become a serious problem, but its impact on our golf game can be dramatic. Even before your round is over, you've likely noticed how stiffness and fatigue negatively impact your performance.

The game of golf can help you live a happier and healthier life by forcing you to pay attention to your physical condition. Rather than waiting six months to address a problem, you'll notice right away when your body isn't responding the way you expect.

Keep this in mind when practicing golf: don't push yourself until you're exhausted, as I used to. Limit the number of skills you try to practice in one session, and limit the time and energy you spend on it. The most effective practice gets your muscles moving sufficiently while leaving enough energy for self-healing and recovery. As I've stated already, recovery is an active process. If you drain all your energy, it will take your body longer to recover than if you keep something in reserve.

Ilchi Posture for Correcting Body Imbalances

I call the following technique "Ilchi Posture." It's extremely simple, but it incorporates the essence of self-healing in two ways: concentration and breathing. Do these exercises immediately following the relaxation and energy-charging routine outlined previously.

Simply lie on your back with your legs extended. Make fists and point the index fingers on both hands. This is the meaning of *ilchi*: one finger pointing the way. Keep pointing your index fingers as you stretch your arms above your head as far as you can, making your whole body feel taller and longer. If stretching your arms above your head feels difficult, adjust your posture by separating your arms farther to the sides until they can relax on the floor.

Ilchi Posture works because it aligns your body, letting energy flow more naturally. If you have imbalances in your spine or muscles, you'll easily identify them through this posture. Have someone check the symmetry of your arms and legs while you practice. They'll see right away if one arm is stiffer than the other or if your body is tilted to one side.

How can you apply the Ilchi Posture? Here's where you start to use the power of your mind. In Ilchi Posture, you can bring awareness deep into your body with each breath. As you breathe in, notice the stretch in your chest, shoulders, and back. As you breathe out, relax more deeply into the posture. This subtle activity is the essence of self-healing. Pay attention to the details rather than focusing on big movements.

As you inhale, feel precisely where your body holds tension. Is it tighter on your right or your left side? At what point do you start to notice resistance when you inhale? The activity of breathing, combined with careful attention, transforms a seemingly static posture into an active practice of self-healing. You'll release stress and tension, calm your mind, and find a sense of centeredness. After a few minutes, your body alignment will naturally improve.

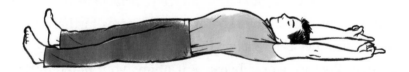

Longevity Walking for Calming Body and Mind

There is an "arms race" of sorts in golf, as equipment becomes more advanced and players hit the ball farther, courses become longer, and riding in golf carts becomes the norm. Walking an entire round is rare on many courses, and impossible on others. And yet, walking is one of the traditional aspects of golf that's most beneficial for mind and body.

If you take no pleasure in walking the golf course, breathing fresh air in the warm sunshine, why not just use a golf simulator? "Golfers, walk on the course whenever you get a chance. Your heart and your brain will thank you for it." This is the thought that 102-year-old golfer Jongjin Lee planted deep in my head. I've always liked walking for pleasure and exercise, but I have tried to walk more on the golf course since playing a round with Lee.

I highly recommend walking on the golf course whenever you have the chance. This produces a variety of benefits. First, it provides a significant amount of good exercise. It also helps you appreciate the course and get a feel for how each hole is designed—and if you're carrying your own bag, you'll be inspired to reduce the number of clubs you take. As an added bonus, you'll do less damage to the course by walking. And finally, walking can be an excellent form of meditation.

Specifically, I want to promote what I call Longevity Walking. This is a simple but powerful technique that can help revitalize your body and calm your mind, no matter what's going on around you. Energetic children step with their bodies leaning forward as if they're about to fall, pressing with the balls of their feet. The older we get, though, the more we tend to tilt our bodies slightly backward or bend our upper body with hunched shoulders and back as we walk. Longevity Walking helps to transform an old step back to a young step.

Stand comfortably with your shoulders and chest open and your back straight. Focus on increasing the distance between your solar plexus and your belly button to help straighten your back and lift your chest. In that posture, lean forward slightly, only about one or two degrees. You're tilting your whole body, not bending at the waist. When you do this, you'll feel your brain's attentiveness increasing. Tiny differences in angle create big differences in brain arousal.

On the sole of each foot, about a third of the way down from the toes, is the acupuncture point called the *yongchun*. In Korean, yongchun means that life energy is rising like water from a spring. Keeping your attention on that spot, stand with your toes slightly flexed and feel as if they're gripping the ground.

The 100-Year Golfer

From this position, step lightly with the heel of your foot, really press the ground with the ball of your foot, and continue to step forward, pressing down through the tip of your big toe. It's helpful to imagine using the balls of your feet to press buttons popping out of the ground as you walk. As is widely known through reflexology, the soles of the feet contain nerves that connect with the entire body. That's why evenly stimulating the soles of your feet as you walk has the effect of "massaging" your whole body.

Pay attention to make sure you are walking with your feet in parallel alignment, like the number 11. Walking with the feet turned outward will cause energy to leak out. You'll be better balanced, and your upper and lower back will expand better, if you walk with both feet pointing in the same direction. Let your arms swing naturally. It's even better if you walk with a smile on your face! In a state of high brain arousal, a refreshing stimulation is sent to your whole body, and rhythmic stimulation is transmitted to your brain whenever the center of your foot touches the ground. You'll feel a pleasant bounce, as if you have springs on the bottoms of your feet.

Longevity Walking is similar to the gait of a cat in some ways—you take one light step at a time instead of plodding along heavily. It's an elegant gate, pleasant and centered. To walk like this, your body should be relaxed, free of tension. Relax and lower your center of gravity into your feet as you do when swinging a club. Try to feel where your center of gravity is: neck, lower back, legs, or feet. Walk with awareness of your body's center of gravity shifting left and right as each foot touches the ground.

Be mindful of the tempo of your walking. Walking even a little too fast for your personal condition will cause your energy consumption to increase, tiring you out and making you lose the rhythm of your breathing. As you walk, imagine earth energy rising from the bottoms of your feet up along your legs, passing your knees and hip joints, and collecting in your lower belly. Focus on gently pressing the center of your feet into the ground with each step. This will cause any fire energy that has been driven upward by stress to sink into the soles of your feet, calming your mind and activating Water Up, Fire Down energy circulation.

Longevity Walking is a kind of "reset" gait. As you walk, you can check your body and mind and restore the centeredness and balance that you have lost. On your way to play your next shot, rather than ruminating over your score on the last hole, simply walk—feeling the soles of your feet, looking up at the sky, taking in the trees. You'll be able to find peace of mind and strength.

You can learn a lot about a course through your feet. The condition of the turf, the angle of the slope, the softness of the greens—all these things can be felt through your feet. Develop sensitivity and awareness in your feet, and your game will certainly benefit.

One example of using your feet is the aim-point putting method. Aim-point has the player assess the slope of the green by "feeling" it with her feet and then applying this feeling to the line of the putt. Obviously, the better your ability to feel, the better you will putt.

Walking is a great example of how the mind impacts our physical experience. When we walk mindfully, we can recharge our bodies and focus our attention. If we walk stiffly and without awareness, though, it's more likely that we'll feel drained and scattered when it comes time for our next shot.

In our hyper-competitive, statistics-obsessed modern world, it's easy to forget the benefits of something as simple as going for a walk. When we primarily take our pleasure from shooting a lower score or hitting the ball farther than others, we tie ourselves to an experience that is going to be frustrating more often than not.

I'd encourage you to think of your time spent walking as a moving meditation—a time to release your worries, exercise your body, and connect with nature. With this mindset, you are guaranteed to feel that you have benefited from the time you've spent golfing, regardless of your score.

The Importance of Mental and Emotional Self-Care

S elf-care is essential to help deal with the physical stress of practicing and playing golf. Physical self-care can be directed toward recovery, injury prevention, and performance enhancement. You may go to the gym to strengthen your core and back muscles to prevent injury on the course. After playing, you may want to spend 20 to 30 minutes doing a set of relaxation and stretching exercises to help your body recover. Or, you can focus on performance-enhancing exercises that help you hit the ball farther and straighter. All of this is probably familiar to you, and all of it can be considered self-care.

I've suggested a couple of unconventional exercises for physical self-care in the previous pages, but I also want to talk about something that might be unfamiliar to you yet is equally important. In golf, as in any endeavor, mental and emotional self-care is essential for your success.

What is mental and emotional self-care? Contrary to how it might sound, it's not just about making yourself feel better.

Basically, this kind of self-care is rooted in understanding how the human brain works.

In golf, as in life, we're constantly challenged with new obstacles and opportunities. Each hole tempts us with a new image of success. When things go the way we hoped they would, we feel joy and peace. When things go contrary to our hopes and dreams, we naturally feel frustrated or disappointed.

Anyone who plays golf regularly will have developed their own relationship with these ups and downs that occur over time—month by month, round by round, and moment by moment. There are two basic mindsets with which we can address this rollercoaster of emotions. One is addiction; the other is self-care.

Many people joke about being "addicted" to golf. It's true— many golfers display addictive behavior. They're impatient, irrational, and highly motivated to achieve a specific kind of "high." Gamblers sometimes exhibit similar tendencies when they're addicted to the thrill of winning, even though most of the time they end up losing more than they win.

Choosing to practice self-care is one of the most effective ways to interrupt the downward spiral of addictive behavior in golf and in life. When you actively incorporate self-care into your life, you break the cycle of desire and reaction that characterizes addiction.

Instead of being primarily focused on results and how they make you feel, self-care brings your focus to the value of the experience itself. By taking action to appreciate the experience, you naturally cultivate a sense of gratitude and purpose. Self-care is not only about getting the results that will make you happy; it's about creating happiness that you can utilize in your practice, independent of the day-to-day results.

Here are a few great self-care tips to incorporate into your golf routine:

- **Don't rush.** Whether you're in the parking lot, at the first tee, driving your cart, or walking down the fairway, take your time. This doesn't mean you should be slow. You may play more quickly when you focus on moving at a relaxed pace on the course.

- **Recite an affirmation** at some point in your routine. Whether it's when you're taking off a glove, taking a practice swing, reading a putt, or marking down your score, add a positive self-care message to your routine. Here are my favorites:

  » My body is not me, but mine.
  » My mind is not me, but mine.
  » I play golf with joy.
  » I have a natural swing.
  » I'm deeply connected with myself and with my golf.
  » I love my golf and my golf loves me.
  » I will play golf until I'm 100 years old.

To increase the energy of my affirmations, I often add these words at the end: "Yes, I am" or "Of course, I am" or "Yes, I do" or "Of course, I do."

- **Don't cheat.** If you've put yourself in a position where you need to lie about your results to yourself or others, you're not playing the game in a healthy way.

- **Accept mistakes maturely.** They're going to happen. Keeping your equanimity in the face of mistakes helps prevent the effects of stress and negative emotions.

- **Be kind to your playing partners,** even if they're not able to do the same. How you treat your partners affects your own mental and emotional health even more than that of the people around you. Being kind to your partners ultimately means being kind to yourself.

- **Take a moment to appreciate nature.** Being in nature has proven to be its own therapy and is one of the inherent benefits of golf. Letting your attention rest on the natural beauty around you can prepare your mind for the next shot.

These are some simple examples of self-care. As you practice and play, you can cultivate your own way to maintain a mental and emotional state that is balanced, focused, and positive.

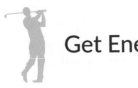

Get Energy from Nature

Connecting with nature is a powerful way to bring self-care and self-healing to your golf. The golf course itself is an artificial construct, but nature is there within it. You can see the green grass and trees, encounter the wide-open sky, feel the warm sunshine and cool breeze, and hear the chirping of birds and grasshoppers.

When I'm in Sedona, I usually play at Seven Canyons Golf Club. Surrounded by towering red-rock mountains, green juniper trees, and the clear blue sky, this course is famous for its beauty. I usually play early in the morning—it's not uncommon for me to have the first tee-time of the day. I like the cool, refreshing energy before the desert sun heats the atmosphere. Plus, it's quiet at that hour, so I can better hear the songs of birds filling the golf course. The wet grass sometimes makes things difficult on the first hole, but that's more than offset by the beauty of the morning, which feels divine.

I like to walk, but I have to ride a cart to reach the fifth tee at Seven Canyons because it's at the top of a very steep hill. I still remember the first time I stood on that tee; every exclamation I knew came pouring from my mouth. I could see the entire course below me, and I felt as if I'd been lifted from the ground to touch the sky. Even now, I feel awe when I overlook the fifth hole, high in the mountains, with the blue sky above me and the surrounding red rocks seeming almost within reach.

When I first began to play golf, everything on the course felt like an enemy barring my way. Narrow fairways and undulating greens, deep bunkers and menacing water hazards—all looked like painful obstacles. Now, though, the golf courses I often visit feel like old friends to whom I can open my heart without hesitation. With friends like that, I can sit in silence without any awkwardness; just seeing them makes me feel good. In the same way, there are times when I get strength merely by going to the golf course, regardless of how my game turns out. A water hazard seems heartless when it swallows my golf ball, but it looks lovely when I see its surface sparkling under the midday sun, and I feel grateful for it.

You won't notice nature all around you at the golf course when you're focused solely on your score. Don't look only at the ball. Take a break sometimes to look at the sky and water, and listen to the sounds of the birds and the wind, recharging yourself with energy from nature. Escaping from dreary city surroundings, enjoy the feelings of liberation and freedom that come from playing in the embrace of nature. You can feel nature in your golf swing, too, not just in natural objects. Relax and sense the weight of the clubhead, watch and feel its gravity and centripetal force. Experience the very laws of nature, trust that they are supporting your golf game, and send your ball flying with the powerful swing you've been imagining.

Golf Is Fun Even after Knee Replacement

By Reinette Krajci
62-year-old woman, New York, USA, three years of golf experiencerience

After working as a schoolteacher, I retired three years ago and started playing golf. There are a lot of good public golf courses around me. I play nine holes with my husband every day and 18 holes once every week or two. I do it even in winter, as long as it's not raining, or the temperature isn't falling below 40°F.

I started Body & Brain Yoga practice eight years ago, and it's helped me a lot to stay healthy and have more fun playing golf. It's improved my strength, flexibility, and balance and has enhanced my range of motion in my back and torso. I use Body & Brain Yoga practice as a warmup before a tee shot. When I arrive at the golf course, I first do some light walking; then I do a 10-minute routine for stretching my major muscles and joints. I regularly do exercises to develop my balance and relax my neck, shoulders, wrists, and hands. I pay special attention to my wrists. It's easy to get hurt if you hold the club too tight. But wrist exercises give you a more comfortable, more flexible grip.

I replaced both my knees with artificial joints at the age of 52. The surgery went well, and my range of motion was also good, but I started Body & Brain Yoga practice and could kneel without any worries. I had no problem squatting down on the green to check my putting line. My bone density increased from 5.2 to 5.4 percent. My doctor gave a thumbs up and asked what I'd been doing. I think it might have been due to my yoga training and golf.

I'm not that good at golf, but I'm not that bad either. I've been having a lot of fun. Recently, I've often played rounds with other female golfers. Now, I'm focusing on increasing accuracy and avoiding injury in my golf game. I pay special attention to warming up enough before the tee shot.

Meditation, breathing, and exercises for training my core have taught me to focus and maintain my balance. Even if things are crazy around me, I'm able to go within, maintaining composure and concentrating on what I have to do right now: put the ball in the hole.

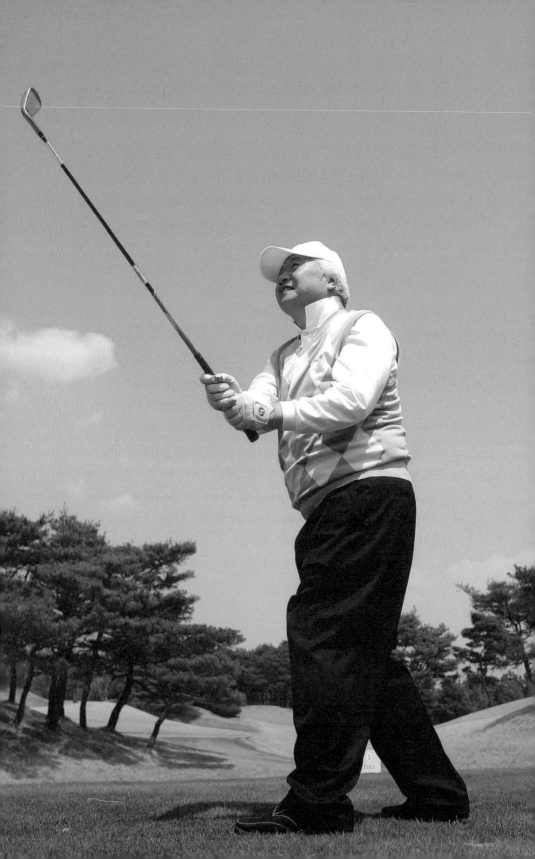

Consciousness Determines the Quality of Your Golf Experience

Growth Stages of Golf

Numerous sayings emphasize the importance of mindset in the game of golf. This game is commonly said to be 30 percent physical and 70 percent mental. Golf legend Jack Nicklaus has even said that the sport is 90 percent mental and 10 percent swing. But this applies only to the pros and seasoned golfers who've been at it a long time. It's quite the opposite in the beginning when you're just learning. At that point, golf is more like 70 percent physical and 30 percent mental.

You must first use your body to learn the basic skills and develop the senses required for golf. You must swing a golf club 10,000 times before your swing feels natural. As with many things in life, there is no substitute for physical practice in golf. Once you've learned the basics and gotten used to the swing, then the more you play, the more you understand how your mind affects golf and the more it becomes a mental game.

There's a principle of Sundo that can explain the developmental stages of golf in terms of energy—*Jungchoong, Kijang, Shinmyung.* Translated literally, this means that when your vital energy is full, then your heart energy matures and your spiritual energy brightens. It means that our energy goes from physical fullness through emotional maturity to mental and spiritual brightness. It also refers to an ideal energy state in which the body, mind, and spirit move as one rather than acting separately.

Physical Development of Golf

The first stage, Jungchoong, refers to the process of acquiring energy by physically training the body. In particular, it's vital to strengthen the dahnjon, the energy center of the lower abdomen. In golf, the Jungchoong stage is about building the physical foundation to practice and play the sport. It's a process of faithfully learning and practicing your grip on the golf club, your setup posture, and the basics of your swing. Your body will develop these skills only with repetition, and only if you do your best to concentrate on each small, seemingly trivial movement without skimping or skipping. You can't make a swing your own unless you learn it with your body through practice, no matter how many YouTube videos you watch or how many golf books you read. Endless repetition is necessary to reach a certain level of performance in any sport—or with any musical instrument—not just golf.

When learning or changing your golf swing, get your body used to the new movements first. To change an arm angle even a few degrees, someone who has developed their swing through years of practice must employ muscle patterns, forces, and senses that are different from what they've been using. They have to be patient and keep repeating the new motions until their muscles remember the new patterns of movement and energy at an unconscious level.

Golf is a sport that requires a lot of practice. Even professional golfers practice constantly and get regular coaching to improve and maintain their skills at a certain level. When I play, I'm often asked by younger golfers, "How do I relax?" and "How do I get rid of my anxiety?" Each time, I teach them several of the meditation and breathing techniques I've introduced in this book. But in fact, practice is what's most important. Unless you practice, you won't have many opportunities to use the various mind-body training techniques I've included. Jungchoong Golf—swinging with a balanced posture, the body comfortable, relaxed, and centered in its abdominal core—is created through steady practice.

Golf for Emotional Maturity

Once you've mastered the basics of golf and have created a good foundation, it's time to pay attention to golf at the Kijang level. In the stages of energy development, Kijang refers to emotional maturity and balance. In Sundo, this means you practice keeping the energy center in your chest, your heart, balanced and open.

It used to sound strange to talk about emotions in sports, but now it's widely known how much emotion impacts the performance of athletes. Emotions are not just felt in the head, nor are they limited to the heart. Feelings affect every cell of our bodies. Powerful emotions can paralyze our arms and legs, take our breath away, and make our head spin. They can make our bodies ice cold and burning hot. From this perspective, emotion management is also body management.

As a golfer, you're probably aware that slight changes in your emotions can affect your body. First-tee jitters can make your head spin, your back tight, and your legs weak. On the other hand, sinking a long birdie putt can put you at ease on the next hole, making your body feel light and relaxed, flexible, and strong. But when you're dealing with the frustration of a bad shot, a bad bounce, or even an inconsiderate playing partner, being able to handle your emotions can be the difference between playing your game and falling apart.

The ability to recognize and recover from anxiety or nervousness, an attitude that lets you calm down and start again even when the game isn't going your way, a can-do, confident attitude of never giving up, and a strong mindset allowing you to show respect and consideration to your companions and not be shaken by their games—these all reflect mature emotional management.

Emotional management before and after a round is as important as it is during play. How do you prepare before playing golf? Do you feel pleasant tension and excitement even while keeping your body and mind sufficiently relaxed? Or is your body stiff because of pressure to do well or worry that you might repeat the mistakes of the last round? After playing, how do you feel about the results? Are you able to look dispassionately at the inevitable ups and downs of golf with acceptance and good humor? Or do you lose sleep at night because of a missed putt on the 18th hole?

In the stages of energy development, Jungchoong is a prerequisite for Kijang. Just as a boat is swept away by the current unless it's properly anchored, we are staggered by the ups and downs of our thoughts and emotions unless we've developed an energy anchor through Jungchoong. The same goes for golf. Anxiety or nervousness mostly comes from a lack of self-confidence. The surest way to have confidence is to build a solid foundation in the basics and then practice, practice, practice. Training never lets us down, in life or in golf.

Golf for Creativity and Spirit

If you've developed some physical ability and emotional maturity in the game of golf, you can now move on to the next step, Shinmyung. Shinmyung means that your consciousness expands and becomes brighter. In the stages of energy development, Shinmyung is a state in which the brain's potential awakens and your powers of insight, intuition, and creativity are manifested. This isn't being smart as we commonly think of it; rather, it's a state in which you take the lead in your life and positively impact those around you with a bright, clear mind.

Golf can make you happy, or it can make you sad. One moment you may feel elated, the next, utterly depressed. A round of golf has often been described as a microcosm of life. And as in life, every new event creates an opportunity to decide how you want to react.

We all have different body types, temperaments, and golfing experiences. However, there is one powerful force that all golfers can use in the various situations they encounter while playing golf. That force is consciousness.

Consciousness can also be seen as a state of energy. Not a fixed state, it changes many times a day depending on the situation. It goes back and forth across a broad spectrum—from fear, insecurity, anxiety, depression, lethargy, and anger to confidence, courage, joy, love, and peace.

There's bound to be a state of consciousness and energy in which each person generally resides—a domain of consciousness you keep returning to, like a base camp of sorts. We could say that it's the habitual information that dominates our lives. Simply put, it's the pattern of thoughts or emotions that normally influences our choices. Such patterns act both positively and negatively in our lives. They can be divided into two basic types: victim consciousness and master consciousness.

Victim consciousness is characterized by an outward-driven focus. Everything happens because of someone or something. The way I feel is caused by some event—something someone said, or something that happened or didn't happen to me. Victim consciousness doesn't always feel negative; sometimes it may seem quite pleasant and positive, providing a sense of vindication when we fail. But it is fundamentally a state of focusing outside yourself, and ultimately it leads to anxiety, depression, and hopelessness. Why? Because, when you are in a victim's mindset, things always happen to you, not as the result of your own choices. When we think that the cause of our woes is external, we believe that life will never change unless our circumstances—things we cannot control—change.

Master consciousness, on the other hand, is based on an inward-driven focus. It considers the fact that I am largely in control of how I experience life, even if I don't control everything that happens. Naturally this can be challenging to maintain when life presents us with uncomfortable or frustrating situations. Ultimately, though, it can be a source of inspiration and power, providing a strong faith and will to create the life you want.

Thankfully, golf provides a training ground where we can experience these different kinds of consciousness. Many of us golfers have lived long enough to fully appreciate the importance of self-direction coming from a sense of ownership, both in work and in life. We may already have learned this lesson from life, but applying it on the golf course isn't all that easy. For those of us lucky enough to play golf regularly, the game reveals the true nature of master and victim consciousness and presents an opportunity to practice choosing the more beneficial option. If you want to play Shinmyung Golf, allowing your consciousness to shine even when a situation knocks you off your feet, try to take it like a freestanding punching bag—bouncing back to master consciousness, owning your situation, and making the best choices you can.

The Five Attitudes of a Good Golfer

Of course, if you play golf with outward-driven focus, your sense of self-worth will follow the ups and downs of the game. As your sense of self-worth fluctuates, so will your focus and emotions, and you can't expect a good score under those conditions. Even if you take full ownership of your experience, it doesn't ensure that your scores will improve, but at least you can become a golfer who respects yourself and your companions and enjoys playing the game in good health.

Through my own experience and that of the partners who've shared in my golf adventure so far, I've learned five attitudes necessary for becoming a good golfer. If you train yourself in these attitudes, golf will transcend sports to become a Shinmyung journey for cultivating spirit and character.

1. Accept Reality

Although the game is played with a lifeless ball and club, golf itself is a living thing. The state of our bodies, minds, and energy is loaded unaltered into the golf club and ball. Our swing reflects not only our own condition but also the day's sunshine and wind, the condition of the course, and everything in the surrounding environment. That's why each swing and the flight of the ball are never exactly the same. The range of scores is said to be wider in golf than in any other sport. Since the potential differences can be large, this sport requires a flexible, resilient attitude.

Whatever kind of golf you're playing now, accept it as it is without denying it. Whether you can break par or haven't ever broken 100, whether you top the ball or hit a shank, accept it just as it is. Because that's reality. Those who deny reality can never change it.

This doesn't mean you should resign yourself to the way things are, give up, or have a passive attitude. Positive change begins in knowing what you should change. You can't create the change you want while denying your present state. You must honestly accept your golf game for what it is rather than hoping for lucky breaks or unexpected improvement. If your habit of refusing to accept your game gets worse, you may even suffer a mental breakdown, doing things like secretly switching out a ball you've lost out of bounds.

Accepting reality isn't just about checking scores or techniques. You should take a hard look at your physical, mental, and spiritual experience of golf. Do you see yourself easily giving up, despairing, and compromising when you encounter obstacles? Does your greedy desire to win make you secretly interfere with your partner's game or behave in a petty way after losing? Does your desire to do well put unhealthy stress on your body and mind, straining them like a taut rubber band? You need to accept everything honestly. Be grateful and joyful for a consciousness that's able to see all that. No matter what state you're in, you can move on to the next stage when you are aware of and accept your present condition and have faith that you can change it, just as you created it in the first place.

2. Love Yourself

Does this sound familiar? When your game goes well, you feel great, but when it doesn't, you feel pathetic. No matter how much your companions give encouragement, you beat yourself up on the inside while smiling on the outside. In such moments, what we really need is absolute faith in and love for ourselves. Feeling good and proud when our game goes well doesn't require any training since it's only natural. We most need love and belief in ourselves when our game doesn't go as we want, and we feel like giving up. Loving and encouraging yourself also takes training.

Practice encouraging and loving yourself at every moment when you're playing golf. You don't have to break 90, hit it 280 yards, or be a single handicap before you acknowledge and love yourself. Give up the fear that your golf game will stagnate if you recognize and love yourself now. The thought that we can accept and love ourselves only if certain conditions are met impedes our growth in all of life's games, not just in golf. Praise yourself even on days when you're not happy with how your game went, finding things you did well or new things you learned. If the person you love most was learning to play golf for the first time, you'd pat them on the back, encouraging them though they made mistakes, praising them for even small improvements. Commit to loving and cheering yourself on just like that in every round, whether you've been golfing for one week or one hundred years.

3. Be Grateful

In April of 2021, Japan's Hideki Matsuyama became the first Asian-born player to win the Masters. Matsuyama wowed the crowd on his way to winning his first major that Sunday, but it was his caddy, Shota Hayafuji, who probably ended up making the biggest impression. On the 18th hole, after Matsuyama tapped in his final putt, Shota respectfully grabbed the flag, removed his hat, and bowed to Augusta National Golf Course. He said his heart was full of gratitude, and he just wanted to express it. Golfers from all over the world witnessed his beautiful action and were deeply touched. It connected all of us, from PGA Tour players to fans watching at home, with the noble spirit and highest ideals that we naturally seek through golf. In this sublime moment, Shota's expression of gratitude awakened the gratitude within each of us.

"Of course, it's natural to feel grateful for winning the Masters!" you might think. And some may complain, "I can be thankful only if I have something to be thankful for." To such people I often say, "You turn on the light because it's dark, not because it's bright." We can be grateful because we want a fuller, more satisfying game, not only when we're already satisfied.

There is a very simple way to check the condition of your brain on the golf course: Do you have a positive, grateful heart, or are you mired in dissatisfaction and negative thoughts? If you keep complaining or making lame excuses, you've shut off the light in your brain.

Once you make up your mind to be grateful, you'll find plenty to be grateful for. Aren't you thankful for just being able to get out and play golf? You could be grateful to the playing partner or caddy who is out with you, to the workers who maintain the course you're playing, to your golf balls and clubs, even to the wind and sun and fresh air blessing your day.

Those who make good use of the power of gratitude, even after hitting the worst shot of their lives, will be thankful for hitting bottom, since now the only way left is up! Some may sneer at this, calling it the self-consolation of an incompetent golfer. But it's a much better way to use your brain than brooding over a double bogey, giving your companions the feeling that they're playing with a ticking time bomb. Some people blow things way out of proportion when they're feeling a little down; others are grateful even for the small things and express that gratitude. It's a difference in consciousness, not just personality.

Golfers of any skill level can be thankful for being able to make the effort. Keep trying, and there will be times when you're proud of yourself. Those who can encourage and empower themselves when no one cheers them on have bright, clear minds—Shinmyung consciousness. And people who have trained themselves, developing a habit of love and gratitude toward themselves, can positively impact those around them. Their love for themselves grows, expanding into a desire for the good of all, into love and care for others.

4. Keep a Positive Mindset

Previously, I spoke about emotional maturity and balance in the Kijang stage. People commonly talk about trying to "control" emotions. When you reach the Shinmyung stage, you realize that you can also create feelings. You can create your own contentment, joy, and happiness, not stopping at merely calming any anxiety that arises in your mind. Using your mind, you can create new energy. In short, you can change your feelings and mood.

It's natural for negative emotions to come up when something bad happens. But when you face negative emotions, what's important is having the self-awareness to recognize them and the ability to act, immediately changing your energy. In an overly emotional state, you can't create new feelings or change energy because you're too busy reacting. You have to quickly disconnect from negative information and energy to create new energy. Shinmyung is being able to use your conscious mind as it watches your thoughts, emotions, and actions in any situation.

Everyone gets angry and irritated when their shots keep landing in the rough or out of bounds. Instead of outwardly suppressing your boiling anger and pretending that everything's okay, if you're able to observe your situation and yourself dispassionately—laughing and creating your own positive energy—then you've used your mind and consciousness well. You're also proactively using your mind when you use good humor to break the ice with your playing partners, creating a more pleasant atmosphere.

It's like two sides of the same coin; where there's light, there's shadow. We can't hope for golf to be free of shadows. Those who use Shinmyung—a bright consciousness—are not people without any anxiety, worry, or fear, but rather are people who choose light, hope, and positivity even in such situations. Even when facing a challenging environment, people who can discover and learn something helpful without blaming others or their circumstances are Shinmyung Golfers with truly bright minds.

5. Follow Your Conscience

A golfer's character and personality are nakedly exposed on the golf course. You can know a lot about a person when you play a round of golf with them. It can be more rewarding to play with a high handicapper who has good character than a scratch player who is rude or selfish. Playing golf with companions who respect the dignity of the game and have the virtue of humility, people with whom you can share frank discussions about life, is a happy experience that you will long remember.

There is something noble about golf. It demands that you have a thoughtful attitude of respect and consideration for others, while also being strict and disciplined with yourself. Having good character doesn't mean simply following the rules. A person's character becomes apparent naturally, even unintentionally, like a scent coming from a hidden air freshener. It is revealed by each word and every decision, whether made consciously or not.

Golf is a sport without referees, in which players record their own scores, so it frequently tempts players to cheat. Some intentionally move their golf ball to a good spot on the green, while others deliberately falsify their score. Players like this may be able to avoid an immediate crisis or win a close game through these actions, but they lose something more substantial. Abandoning their conscience causes them to lose confidence and pride in themselves. Their minds crumble.

Conscience is the bright mind within us. We each make our own judgments about right and wrong because we have a conscience. We feel discomfort when there's a discrepancy between our words and our deeds, our knowledge and our practice, and we make up our minds to overcome that discrepancy. If you frequently violate your conscience on the golf course, you will inevitably distance yourself from Shinmyung Golf.

"At 70," Confucius confessed, "I could follow the dictates of my own heart, for what I desired no longer overstepped the boundaries of right." If you can follow the dictates of your own heart on the golf course, you have brightly illuminated the divine within you—an achievement worthy of self-praise.

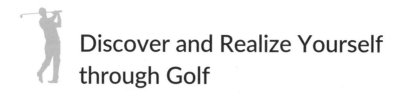

Discover and Realize Yourself through Golf

Golf isn't only about having fun. It also involves toil, discomfort, and suffering. Why do we continue to play golf, enduring all of that? Could it be that we find joy in growing to discover and realize a new self? You can come close to Shinmyung Golf if you make the sport a means for growing through interactions with yourself, your golf partners, and nature, not a mere contest for taking strokes off your game.

If you set a goal for your golf and practice, you'll find that sometimes you succeed in meeting that goal and sometimes you don't. Your game doesn't improve only when you're successful, though. The important thing is that you keep trying and staying with it, one way or another. You can't master your golf skills or change your habits or attitudes on the golf course all at once. It's enough to just practice regularly and truthfully, without being in a rush, and to be happy doing it. When you fail, instead of blaming yourself, it's enough to dispassionately acknowledge the present reality and learn from that experience.

In training to achieve a goal, there is no success or failure. There are only constant challenges and experiences directed toward your golf goals. It's a path of self-directed growth involving neither success nor failure. Knowing your limitations and golfing within them while challenging yourself to expand the boundaries bit by bit—that is the joy of golf.

A beautiful aura surrounds golfers who let their consciousness shine, who aren't dominated by their environment, instead thinking of all circumstances they encounter as a stage upon which to learn and act. When they stand on the golf course close to the age of 100, though their bodies are smaller than before and their steps are slower, their spirits shine through their gentle smiles and bright eyes. They lift their clubs comfortably and make their best swing as smoothly and naturally as they can. Wherever the ball goes, a gentle smile never leaves their lips, and their eyes sparkle, curious about what the next shot might bring. Wisdom for life flows from their lips—words heard sparingly in the silence, pleasant to the ear, long remaining in the heart. This is the picture I'm drawing of the elder golfer who has reached Shinmyung.

Depending on what you think about its purpose, golf can become a spiritual practice for illuminating your mind and cultivating your character. It becomes a steppingstone for growth and endless self-development, an art for creatively expressing yourself. The self you seek through golf is no different from the self looked for by spiritual seekers. Our lives are a process of finding and realizing that self.

In South Korea, older people are sometimes called *eoreushin*. That means someone whose spirit is great and bright, and wise like a god. Not everyone becomes an elder just because they're old. When we meet people whose years of experience have made them strong in spirit, whose wisdom lights up those around them, we call them "elders" out of respect, not as a mere ceremonial title. If you're worn out by life and trapped by prejudice, or if you're petty and selfish even in your 70s or 80s, you just look like an old man or woman. I want to meet many true elders on the golf course, people whose spirits are bright and who have reached the stage of Shinmyung.

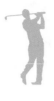

Bowing Meditation— Emptying Yourself and Letting Go of Your Attachments

One method of meditation that helps with Shinmyung Golf, turning golf into a means of character development, is bowing. Many might think of specific religious traditions when you mention bowing, but if you discard such preconceptions, you'll find this universal practice is a wonderful form of exercise and meditation.

Bowing meditation is also a good exercise for establishing Water Up, Fire Down. Since it continually moves the lower body, any energy concentrated in the head sinks into the legs and feet, making the head clearer and the lower body more solid. It centers and balances physical energy and comfortably relaxes the mind.

Bowing meditation involves the very simple movement of bending at the waist, lowering your body to touch your forehead to the floor, and then rising again, repeating this as many times as you want. Stand comfortably with your feet together. Raise your hands in a big circle, bringing your palms together above your head and then lower them, palms still touching, in front of your chest. Bend your upper body

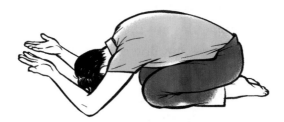

forward and slowly bend your knees, lowering yourself until your knees and then your forehead touch the floor and your buttocks rest on your heels; steady yourself with your hands as needed. Lift your upper body, keeping your buttocks on your heels, and then bring your hands together again, palms touching in front of the chest. Flex and extend your legs, raising your body and returning to the starting posture.

For this exercise, you can complete a set number of repetitions—20, 50, or 100, for example—or a set duration, such as 10 or 15 minutes. If you have bad knees, do the bowing motion slowly. If bowing makes you short of breath, you're doing it too quickly. Catch your breath and then proceed more slowly.

Bowing meditation may seem boring and repetitive at first, superficially involving no significant changes. As you continue bowing, though, you let go of old things, set aside attachments, and learn acceptance instead of resistance. Meanwhile, your body and mind will feel lighter before you know it.

Bowing meditation and golf have similarities in that you always seem to be facing the same challenges without much change, no matter how much you practice, until the moment you discover that you've grown. That's why you keep golfing with faith and hope, despite the unavoidable stress. While experiencing the ups and downs of golf, you never know when you'll realize, "Wow, I'm not who I used to be."

Body lowered, forehead to the ground, you learn that only when you completely accept yourself as you are can you reduce the suffering you feel while playing golf. Raising your body up again, you believe you can continue growing despite all obstacles. After you finish bowing, sit quietly and feel the beating of your heart, your breath coming in and going out, to recover your center and peace of mind. Let love and gratitude for golf fill your heart, and be excited by the thought of playing another round.

I'm Playing the Most Satisfying Game in My 62 Years of Golf

By Jay Odice
76-year-old man, Chicago, USA, 62 years of golf experience

Four years ago, I started learning tai chi at the Body & Brain Yoga center. I also read Ilchi Lee's *I've Decided to Live 120 Years*. I was inspired to design the years I have left, and I'm applying the book's contents to my life. By consistently practicing tai chi and meditation, I've improved my condition and balance, and I've lost 15 pounds without even trying.

Probably the most surprising change was in my golf game. I've played golf for 62 years; in my 20s, I was a single-digit handicap around 6, and I even won some tournaments. I'm 76 now.

My handicap dropped by 4.5 strokes during my last golf season after being the same for almost 10 years. I didn't play golf as much as I used to, and I didn't take any lessons. As I practiced Body & Brain Yoga, my flexibility and range of motion improved noticeably. I do the tapping and stretching I learned at Body & Brain Yoga instead of regular golf warmup exercises, and they are very effective.

The most significant thing was that I started to realize that I could use my brain to get in touch with various parts of my swing. Even though it's just a split second from here to here, I could shift from using force to using energy, and that was a huge shift for me. I had a clearer sense of where I was in the golf swing. Instead of just starting and kind of losing touch, I began to notice where the club was moment by moment. I could tell if I was rushing, or if I was drifting off the ball, or coming down a little steep. I felt like things had slowed down, and I could maintain awareness throughout my swing. This was huge for me. I could notice when I stopped turning because I was getting tired and making adjustments. The result has been that I'm hitting the ball with more confidence and control. Getting in touch with and using the brain to access that ability was an amazing benefit to the game.

You know how your mind gets in the way of your swing when you think too much? It's really being conscious of how to get to an "empty brain." You can still have your best form from your natural experience of swinging without letting the noise get into your head. Everything from the shoulders up is totally relaxed. Before I start my swing, particularly on the drives, I recollect where my swing is, and then I let my body do it without forcing it. It's much more natural.

Even now, I play golf three times a week. I'm still driving the ball 240 to 270 yards. At 76, I'm hitting it longer than I did in my 20s. Of course, part of it is because technology has developed, resulting in better equipment. My goal this year is to become an age shooter by hitting 76 at Chicago's notoriously difficult Blackstone Golf Course.

I look at some of the people I play with. Even in their 70s and 80s, they've got a good game. One of them even shot his age three times this season alone. Two weeks ago, my golf partner was 94 years old. He hit some good driver shots and never hesitated when putting. I also played a bridge game with him. His concentration and energy were great.

But most of them hate trying new things. They'd rather keep doing what they always do. I think my mindset is, "Let's give it a try." If you don't try it for yourself, how can you ever know what it's going to do for you? There's only so much you can understand without trying. On the course, I guess you could say I take this same mindset. Having done Body & Brain Yoga makes me feel like I can find new ways to do things. I feel like I can play each shot in a new way. Maybe I can relax a little more, focus on my lower abdomen, or do some breathing exercises, or I can visualize the shot I want to hit. I can be creative and use my mind and body instead of just forcing it the same way I did before. I have options.

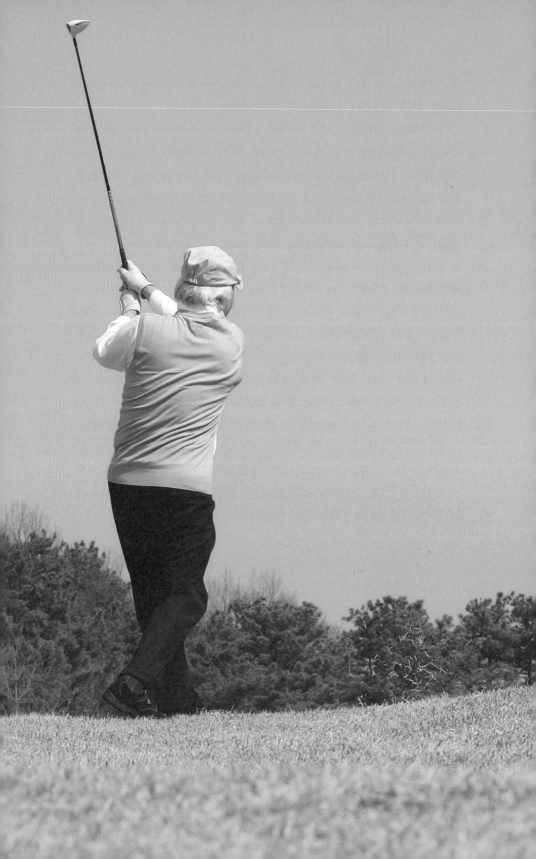

PART 3

Golf and Life

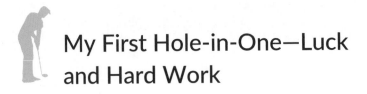

My First Hole-in-One—Luck and Hard Work

About five years after I had started golfing, I got a chance to play during a business trip to Jeju Island in South Korea. The course was beautiful, with a view of Mt. Sanbang and the sea off the city of Seogwi-po.

After some mediocre play, we arrived at the 11th hole with no special feeling. It was a short par 3 about 150 yards long. I stood on the teeing ground, barely able to see the top of the flagpole above the hole because of a hill right in front of the green. The bulging mound looked just like a traditional Korean grave.

I set up with a six iron and swung. The ball shot off with a satisfying thwack. I saw it rising higher than I'd expected, flying over the hill in front of the green and heading toward the flagpole. It fell somewhere out of sight, and I went to pick up the tee.

Suddenly I heard a loud noise coming from the green. People were yelling and waving their hands, and I wondered what all the fuss was about. Only after I reached the green did I realize that my ball was already in the cup. It was my first hole-in-one!

The golf club gave me a hole-in-one cup and a three-day voucher for a nearby luxury hotel. I also bought a good meal for my companions, who were more excited than I was. I was happy, of course, but stunned. I felt awkward, even a little embarrassed, as if I'd brushed aside people much better than I to win an award that I hadn't put much effort into. There were decent single-handicap players among my companions. And at that time, I primarily went to a practice range, making it out onto a golf course only once in a blue moon.

There's something I often heard old-timers say when I was a beginning golfer: luck is 7, skill 3. That means that golf is 70 percent luck and 30 percent skill. I chuckled to myself at that time, thinking, "Does that make any sense? Skill has got to be, like, 70 percent. They just say that to make themselves feel better."

But luck was definitely the deciding factor in my first hole-in-one. My swing did have to be good, of course. But I couldn't even see the bottom of the flagpole, and I hit the ball without knowing the slope of the green around the hole. According to the caddy from the previous group, my ball pitched just beyond the hole cup, stopped for a second, and then rolled down the incline into the cup. I had to acknowledge that forces I couldn't have predicted were at play.

The more I golf, the more my thinking leans toward the 70-30 split between luck and skill. You run across lots of situations that can really be nothing but luck. A ball flies out of bounds, only to bounce off a tree and land happily in the middle of the fairway. You skull a chip and it shoots across the green, only to hit the flagstick and drop into the hole.

On the other hand, sometimes you hit a straight long drive, sending the ball rocketing down the fairway, and you approach with high hopes of getting onto the green in two—only to have them dashed when you find the ball half-submerged in a muddy spot on the fairway. When golfing in the desert of Arizona, there have been times when my ball got stuck in a cluster of impenetrable cactuses or ricocheted off the bone-dry turf into someone's yard, where it joined a growing collection of lost golf balls.

Sometimes it helps to think of *everything* as 70 percent luck, both in golf and in life. That doesn't mean that your effort and capabilities are unimportant. I'm not trying to comfort myself or make excuses about hitting a bad shot or letting an ill-mannered partner interrupt my concentration. And I'm absolutely not saying that your fate is sealed. But I believe those who've found their values and purpose in life create their own destiny. No matter which route you take, if your destination is clear, and you don't forget or give up on it, you will eventually reach that destination, or at least get close to it. Even if you have to overcome obstacles or rest when you get tired, you will eventually arrive at your destination.

I'd like to interpret the 70-30 split this way: "Go all the way with whatever you decide to do, never giving up, but remember that 70 percent of it is a blessing from heaven."

The flow of nature, ever-changing and moving, and the cosmic conditions of space and time—these are luck. That flow acts on individuals, sometimes bringing good fortune, sometimes bad. Luck isn't something we can control. But good fortune rarely comes to those who don't even try. It comes most often to those who do their best.

The more you work, the more your skills improve, and the more your skills improve, the more good opportunities you'll encounter. When you seize promising opportunities, lots of good things happen. The more good things happen, the luckier you'll feel. Seventy percent or more of it will feel like it happened with the aid of heaven or other people. Sometimes it feels like everything good happens automatically, even if I haven't done anything at all. But when I look deeply into such situations, I find that I've actually done a lot of work. Everything just felt like it was going well because I went with the flow, not resisting the space or time of the here and now.

In fact, "I was lucky" is something successful people can say often. Hall of Fame golfer Se-ri Pak says in almost all her interviews, "I was really lucky." Who would think it was luck that got her there? One anecdote gives us some idea of just how hard she practiced. When she was a teenager, her father dropped her off at the practice range in the morning but forgot to go pick her up late into the evening. Realizing this only after he got home, he rushed to the practice range, worried. Se-ri was there, practicing alone until after midnight. "The more you practice, the luckier you are," said golf legend Gary Player. "Fortune favors the prepared," said Virgin Group founder Richard Branson.

"I'm a really lucky person." For me, these words are a comfort, cheering on my brain and keeping the flame of my hope alive. Some days, I repeat these words dozens of times.

On the day I left South Korea and arrived in New York to bring Brain Education and Body & Brain Yoga to the United States, I was robbed at the airport. I lost my bag and all my start-up money, and it all happened in the blink of an eye. I was devastated. Was this a sign that I shouldn't have come to America? Should I go back to South Korea? All sorts of thoughts went through my head.

But I couldn't stop there, halting my path forward in the United States, so I comforted my heartbroken brain by thinking this: "America has given me a special welcoming ceremony. I wonder what great blessings it has in store for me? I'm really lucky. I'm looking forward to the good fortune to come." I decided to think of the $5,000 I'd lost not as money that had been stolen but as my contribution to the city of New York. And I made up my mind to earn a thousand times that in America in the next 10 years.

What seemed like lousy luck at the time became what motivated me, igniting my passion. Whenever things were hard, I'd think about what had happened, pumping myself up. While I had many difficulties, I was able to keep the commitment I'd made to myself in less than 10 years, establishing more than 100 centers teaching Brain Education across America and succeeding with other ventures as well.

Whether we see them as good luck or bad luck, all events we encounter in life are nothing more than growth opportunities when viewed from a long-term perspective. Fundamentally, I don't think there is such a thing as "bad luck." Consequently, there's no reason to blame your luck. We simply need the will and passion to go forward toward our goals and the humility, gratitude, and wisdom to learn and grow through our experiences.

Luck comes and goes. No one can stop the flow of fortune. The incredible Bobby Jones left this famous saying: "In the long run, luck is equal and fair." Trying your best is the way to ensure that luck is on your side, both in golf and in life. Heaven helps those who help themselves, if they stay focused and never give up the goals and purpose they've established. And for those who truly do their best, help comes from the people around them before it comes from heaven.

Golf and life are uncertain. Nothing is predetermined. And while uncertainty can bring us anxiety and pain, at the same time it enriches our lives by making us ever-striving and creative. Isn't golf more fun because you never know what the ball will do on the next shot or how the next round will play out? The next time you play golf, think about how lucky you are, not how unlucky. Many golfers soon forget their good shots yet long remember their bad shots. But people who use their brains well think of it the other way around. Do your best, shot by shot, remembering the good ones and forgetting the bad. Try to think of yourself as really lucky every time you play golf. Even the Fates lack the power to beat those who think of themselves as lucky no matter what happens.

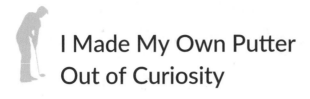

I Made My Own Putter Out of Curiosity

I've practiced putting all by myself, even marking the ball horizontally in thirds and then targeting the top, middle, and bottom. I've also divided it vertically, trying to hit the left, middle, and right. My putting skills didn't improve that much, though. I'd think I had a feel for it one day, only to lose it the next. Then one day, stunned at missing a putt of less than a yard, I thought, "I might as well hit it with my hand."

That night I dreamed I was putting with my hands. Extending my fingers, I touched them to the ground and hit the golf ball with my thumb, as if I were playing marbles. The ball rolled right into the cup! I felt so good that I was probably smiling while dreaming.

I kept thinking of that dream every time I putted. What should I do to putt as if I were using my hands? This line of thinking kept going in my mind, like a snake devouring its tail. The putter has a long, narrow face, but wouldn't I be able to concentrate better if it were a little shorter? I tried putting with a sand wedge, which has a face that's sharper and shorter. It wasn't easy, but I ended up concentrating better, and the balls traveled more accurately. Yet after a few weeks, the sand wedge was no longer satisfactory. It occurred to me that it would be great if the clubface was just the size of a golf ball. I couldn't find a club like that, though.

I finally decided to try making my own putter. When I went to a manufacturer, he asked me to draw a picture of it. After staring at my roughly drawn putter design for a while, he smiled broadly and said, "I can definitely do it." The problem was that the minimum quantity was 300 clubs. The cost was high since we had to create a mold and produce 300 units. I hesitated, but my curiosity wasn't going to quiet down until it had been satisfied. I wanted to try putting with a putter of my own design, and I wanted to confirm whether there was anything to my idea that a short club face might increase putting accuracy. In the end, I made up my mind to put my decision into action.

The club face of the putter I made is just the size of a golf ball, and the back of the head looks like a horseshoe with two thin prongs inside. The result looks vaguely like the hand I had been dreaming of. When I first stood on the green holding the putter I'd designed, my heart pounded with curiosity and anticipation. What was the result? I was super focused at first, so my putts were good; later, though, my putter wasn't any better than any ordinary one. The head was too small, giving it an unstable feeling. After carrying it for several months, I ended up going back to a regular putter.

Don't you wonder what happened to the other 299 putters? When I went to the golf course carrying that putter, everyone—the caddies and my playing partners—stared wide-eyed, asking what it was. They were even more surprised

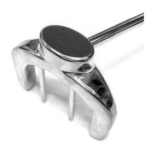
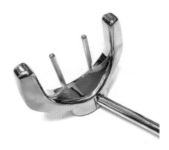

when I told them it was a putter I had designed myself. My putter became the talk of the driving range, and people even waited for me so they could give it a try.

People started saying they wanted my putter. At first, they told me it was "amazing" even though I tried to wave them off, saying that they were experiencing a kind of placebo effect and that it was a failure. But then I started selling them. "Masters," it is said, "don't care about brushes." But we golfers can't shake off the delusions and temptations of a new weapon. So far, I've switched putters more than a dozen times, from expensive, well-known brands to clubs purchased out of curiosity at the neighborhood Walmart. I gave some of the putters I made to close golfing friends, but most I sold. Now only a few are left. At least I recouped the cost of production, so it wasn't a losing business.

You can't really call my putter experiment of 15 years ago a total failure. Since then, I've realized that inventions are

The 100-Year Golfer

nothing special. If you observe with interest and curiosity and find a way to make anything more convenient, more beautiful, or newer, it can be considered an invention. "If you need something, find it; if you can't find it, make it." With this thought in mind, I've developed the habit of trying anything when I get an idea. Thanks to my putter-making experience, I was able to turn other ideas into actual products. This was a great help, as I was able to develop the Belly Button Healing wand, which I designed for gut health; the Bird of the Soul essential oil for meditation, to refresh the brain; and a variety of products using Dendropanax plants, which I used to experiment on myself.

In my life so far, I've started many things that seemed beyond my personal abilities. I've had lots of failures but have been able to accomplish most of the things I thought were truly important. What helped me was this thought: "Find what you need, and create what you can't find." I realize that what has supported me in my life, more than the knowledge I learned in school, is my experience of asking and answering my own questions, along with the power to respect and love myself in that process.

"Find what you need, and create what you can't find." This applies to more than just objects or businesses. Anyone can "invent" the life they want if they have this philosophy. There's nothing that says you must live in the world in a set way. You don't necessarily have to play golf that way, either. Life is about constantly asking who you are and what you want, and finding a way to follow through on the answers you get. If you can't find a way, then make one.

It's easy to walk a well-trodden path. But to realize a dream, sometimes you have to blaze a trail where there isn't one, and you may have to go it alone—giving everything you've got, going against the current, and turning your back on the pathways taken by everyone else.

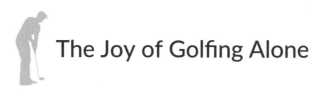

The Joy of Golfing Alone

Golfing alone is so unpopular that there's a joke about it among South Korean golfers: playing 18 holes by yourself is one of the dire punishments of hell. It's often impossible to do so on golf courses in South Korea, because you generally have to create a group of four and are accompanied by a caddy.

In the United States, though, a caddy won't accompany you unless you specifically request one. Many public golf courses don't have caddies at all. And quite often you see people golfing alone. I have many golfing friends in South Korea but only a handful in Arizona or in New Zealand. As a result, I often play alone. I generally golf early in the morning, so I'm frequently the first to tee-off, and there are times when I'm the only person on the wide-open golf course until the next group arrives.

It's sometimes boring when you play by yourself, since you have no one to talk to. You don't have the fun of shouting, "Good shot!" and applauding when your partners do well. Golfing alone, though, has its own pleasures. You can be entirely immersed in your game without being conscious of others. Your problems and shortcomings are more apparent when you focus like that. You feel great when you find solutions and make a good shot after relentless effort. The sense of immersion you get when you focus your energy into each shot without interruption brings great satisfaction and joy. It's rewarding when your game develops, when you feel the improvement brought about through concentration and immersion.

Scores don't mean much when you're golfing by yourself. Sometimes I place and hit two balls, and sometimes I hit the ball five or six times until I'm happy with the shot. When I'm really immersed in the game, I go with the flow, playing rapidly without stopping at all. Time flies on days like that, but I don't even realize it. Playing alone also has the advantage of being quick, with a round taking less than two hours.

One of the pleasures of playing golf alone is enjoying nature more. Sometimes I encounter the sunset when I golf in the late afternoon in Sedona. The sun puts on a spectacle, dyeing the red-rock mountains a golden orange before painting the skies scarlet. Looking up into such a sky, I'm deeply moved, my whole body trembling. I get the feeling that the brilliant colors and lights of nature are penetrating every cell in my body. In those moments, the putt I just missed doesn't matter at all. Nature in all its beauty awakens the pure life within me. I feel the peaceful, complete life inside me, leaving nothing to add or subtract. I want to share the life energy pulsating in me with more people and use it for better things. Welling up like a spring of water, a desire rises in me—a hope for the health, happiness, and peace of all life in the universe.

In moments of deep communion with nature around us, we encounter nature within us. Whole and beautiful, unadorned, nature revives within. Nature and we become one, the boundary between us vanishing. What fills our hearts in such moments is gratitude. We are unconditionally grateful. I'm thankful for being alive now, at this moment. I'm just thankful for everything that has brought me to this moment, regardless of how my golf game went today.

If you have the opportunity, take time to play golf alone. Immerse yourself completely in a game all your own. If it's hard to do that on the golf course, try focusing on the driving range with that mindset. You can concentrate and immerse yourself in anything if you like it, if it's fun, or if it feels meaningful. In immersion, you'll feel a oneness between your work and yourself, between your play and yourself. Such oneness is its own reward, bestowing happiness and joy, and it brings growth and development to everything we do.

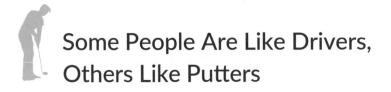

Some People Are Like Drivers, Others Like Putters

"The more I play golf," said golf commentator Henry Longhurst, "the more I think about life, and the more I look at life, the more I think about golf." Any golfer can relate to this.

Golf is often compared to business as well as to life. Like someone running an organization or business, you need goals and strategies in a round of golf. You must efficiently manage all your resources, exhibit the ability to deal with crises, and choose and focus well.

Many CEOs in South Korea, when hiring new talent, intentionally play a round of golf with applicants because the sport reflects a person's character like a mirror, showing what they're made of. Of course, it's not how well the person plays golf that's being scrutinized; it's the person's mindset, integrity, manners, and resilience.

If you're a leader, you'll put a great deal of devotion and effort into finding and developing good talent. Work is ultimately done by people. While the time may have arrived when artificial intelligence is replacing human labor, important planning and decisions ultimately and inevitably pass through human beings. People sometimes can be a headache, but in the end, they are our strength and hope.

Choosing and using golf clubs on the course is a lot like selecting and employing talent in business. Each of the 14 golf clubs has its own purpose. How your game goes will vary greatly depending on which club you use and how you use it. That's why pros aren't allowed to ask which club another player is using during a round.

You need many different clubs to play golf. Similarly, work requires many talented people with different strengths. An organization needs people who take the lead, pioneer new projects, and boldly face challenges—like drivers. Middle managers are like irons, bridging the gap between initiation and the detailed finishing work. It's also important to have people who are reliable, willing to do the "dirty" work and clean up mistakes, like a wedge. And lastly, an organization needs someone who will take responsibility for the precise result, put the finishing touches on the project with sensitivity and relentless attention to detail—putting the ball in the cup like a putter. It's difficult to say that any golf club is best, since each has its own purpose—and so it is with people. If I had to pick, though, I'd like to keep talented, putter-like people close to me.

There's a saying, "Drive for show, putt for dough." In my experience, you can take a risk when deciding on someone to play the role of a driver but not when choosing someone to act as a putter. In the decisive moment when the success or failure of a venture is on the line, you have no choice but to entrust the work to a putter-like person you can rely on.

Even if your distance is short, you can save your game if you have good putting skills, but no matter how much distance you get, you can't produce good results if your putting skills are lacking.

To me, a putter-like person is capable, trustworthy, and reliable. She feels responsible for work no one asked her to do, attends to critical details no one else notices, and focuses until the end. Comparing this to golf, if you're skilled enough to hit a drive 300 yards or more but lose focus when it comes to the short game, you can't be a good leader. My heart goes first to those who do their best regardless of their limitations, who take full responsibility, and who put the integrity of the company or community first in any situation.

In Jim Collins' book *Good to Great*, now a classic in the fields of management and leadership, the author presents five levels of leadership. Competent level-four leaders produce great results with strong charisma and incredible drive but tend to think egocentrically at crucial moments, while great level-five leaders go beyond their egos, knowing how to put the whole before themselves.

In critical moments, you may be tempted to choose personal profit over good faith and honesty. When you accept loss to uphold your core principles, however, your choice shows that you possess a spirit of true leadership. I think a great leader is one who—like a wise golfer—positions each person in a right place with a clear sense of the overarching goal, no matter what kind of distractions or temptations may stand in the way.

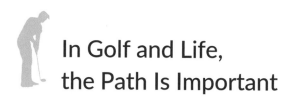

In Golf and Life, the Path Is Important

Anyone who faithfully learns the basics of the golf swing and practices consistently can find a swing path that's right for their body, though some will be faster and some slower. The swing is a motion that obeys physical laws, including gravity and centrifugal force. You can play a satisfying game with your consistent swing if you don't deviate from the best motion your body now allows. The problem is that this principle, which sounds so simple, isn't easy to put into practice.

In most cases, greed or anxiety is why people miss shots even when they possess a good swing. On days when you're driving the ball well, it would be great if you could just maintain a relaxed tempo, but greed creeps up and pushes you to try for more distance. Then, without even realizing it, you tense your body, rush your downswing, sway, cast, etc. . . . and ultimately mess up your shots.

If you struggle with your short game, normally you'd be happy just to hit the green in regulation when you're within 100 yards. But on days when you're feeling really good, you might decide to take dead aim at every flag. If you're not used to this kind of pressure, though, you're more likely to duff or top the ball and have it end up nowhere near the green. Jealousy and anxiety may also arise when a playing partner hits an incredible drive. Even though you've been doing well so far, you may suddenly lose confidence in your swing, or thoughts may flood your head and make you attempt a crazy swing. In other words, greed or jealousy can ruin your swing.

Even after making up your mind to focus on refining your own swing path and not imitate others, greed sometimes catches you like a cold during the change of seasons. No one is entirely free from this pattern—pro or amateur. After winning the U.S. Open, Grand Slam champion Inbi Park confessed to getting queasy just looking at the grass, for fear of failure. That's why golf is best viewed as a lifelong study and as a form of self-discipline for mastering your own mind.

As a sport that requires us to find and continue to hone a swing path that's right for our own bodies, golf is really like life. We strive to discover our life's path our own way in the journey of life that gives us joy and satisfaction.

Golf would be extremely difficult if you had no basic swing path and if you had to use a completely new swing every time you played. The same goes for life. Everyone faces numerous choices in life, and we all need something to serve as a guide each time, like a map or guidebook. This is provided by principles and philosophies. You can continue to trace your path through life only if you have principles and a life philosophy. Principles and philosophies give direction to our lives and keep us from being overwhelmed by life's many choices. When we have standards of value, we're less dominated by moods and emotions. And we're better able to recover any balance lost when we encounter stormy seas on our voyage through life.

In golf, even after we've developed a swing path, we may deviate from it because of our desire to beat others, our wanting to show off, and our doubts and anxiety about our own ability. In the same way, having principles and a philosophy for life doesn't mean we always stay on our life's trajectory. Sometimes we ignore the principles and philosophy we've committed ourselves to follow, and sometimes we lack the drive to follow through on our ideals. These moments are like missed shots on the golf course. Our swing has path, but we have deviated from proper form.

What should you do when you miss shots because you keep deviating from your swing path? The more you try to change and correct your swing during a round, switching to this and that form, the more off-kilter you'll be. At times like this, you need to empty your mind and return to your natural swing with humility, going back to the basics of golf and beginning again from there.

When you think you're staggering through life, empty your heart and return to the basics rather than trying to find and learn more. What kind of person do I want to be, and how do I want to live? What are the most important values and principles in my life? Only by going back for answers to these things can we find direction for our next steps.

You can swing consistently in golf only if your axis of rotation is well fixed. In life, too, you can go your own way with your own tempo and rhythm, without dancing to someone else's tune, only if you have core values that act as an unshakable center.

This doesn't mean you should spend your whole life golfing with the same swing. Your swing is a lifelong study, something you improve little by little, making it clean and consistent, perfecting it until it's all your own. You don't live tracing only a single path in life either. You repeatedly draw arcs large and small. Sometimes you get greedy, as if over-swinging, applying too much force. Sometimes you start out well but end in regret, unable to finish things satisfactorily—like when you rush your downswing and end up hitting it fat or thin. Sometimes, if you change your occupation and the people you share your life with, it's like starting from scratch with a completely new swing. Things may seem to get worse before they get better.

But if you look at the big picture in life, you'll see that deep in your heart you've always wanted one path. You want a life that gives you true inner satisfaction, a life of expressing and realizing your values to your heart's content. Like experimenting with various swing techniques to get the ball more consistently on the green, you may poke your head in different places, glancing down different roads in life, until you find your own method—something that brings your soul peace and stability.

If you know what you truly want and feel that you've lived to accomplish it without regret, you'll be satisfied with your life, no matter how trying it may have been. But you'll feel empty if you've lived without knowing what it is you really want, or if you've set aside your true purpose for lesser priorities, no matter how much you've accomplished or how much others are applauding your triumphs. We feel genuine satisfaction in golf and in life only if we follow our own path, going with our own rhythm and timing. Develop these qualities, above all else, and you will be on your way toward finding your perfect swing.

The Back Nine Holes of My Life

In a round of golf, you'll have holes where you lose a ball out of bounds, but you'll also have holes where you save par after making a miraculous up-and-down out of a deep bunker. Whether in golf or in life, we're given many opportunities. It's vital that we keep trying, never giving up; the game isn't over until you've taken your final shot.

We golfers like comparing golf to life, and in a round of golf, each of the 18 holes can be likened to a moment in life. When I was around 60 years old, I thought that I had finished 12 of my life's 18 holes and that I should be preparing for the home stretch. At 67, though, I started thinking differently. It was then that I began the Earth Village Project in New Zealand. The great dream and hope I felt for this project made me realize I had only finished the ninth hole, the front nine of my life. I was literally just past halfway. I wrote the book *I've Decided to Live 120 Years* around that time.

Early on, during the first three holes of my round—youth and adolescence—I was confused and full of dissatisfaction, feeling like I'd been dragged into a game I didn't want to play. I was resentful about someone or something bringing me into the game of life without my consent, a game that was no fun because I didn't know its meaning or purpose.

At the age of 30, I realized the value and goal of my life and established my purpose. I found my path, the trajectory of my life. When I attached the subtitle "Saving Myself, My People, and Humanity" to my first book, *Dahnhak*, which I wrote at the age of 35, the publisher suggested that it was ostentatious, and I should change it. But I held my ground, insisting that I wouldn't publish the book otherwise, and so I ended up getting it published with the subtitle. Even now, I firmly believe that the way to save ourselves and the planet is for everyone to discover their true value and live with confidence, creativity, and a noble purpose. Of all the things people can do, I think this has the most power for changing the world.

That was the belief I held when I started teaching mind-body training to a man suffering from paralysis in a park in a small town in South Korea. From that beginning, I eventually opened centers nationwide to teach Brain Education and established a university and research institute for studying the practical use of the brain.

Leaving South Korea behind, I passed through a difficult pioneering phase in the United States and arrived at what was about the fifth hole of my life, in Arizona—where I encountered my first hole-in-one. Many amazing things happened in Sedona, and thanks to the blessings of nature and the good friends and supporters I met there, I spent my 50s spreading Brain Education from that home base to more than 10 countries around the world.

In my mid-60s, I went to New Zealand searching for nature and new work to inspire me. There I discovered a heart-pounding new dream: creating Earth Village, an eco-friendly community in the beautiful natural environment of New Zealand, and a school for developing Earth Citizens who embrace humanity, nature, and the world. And I decided to live to 120 years, wanting to achieve that dream and contribute more to making a world where everyone finds their own self-worth.

Everyone encounters a heart-pounding dream at least once or twice in life. However, experiencing hardships, your heart sometimes stops racing and you become frustrated, feeling like you'll never be able to dream again. Many times, I've wondered whether I'd hit my limit—in life and in golf. But no matter how old we are or how many emotional wounds we carry, pure passion and hope remain inside us. Our hearts beat again the instant we recover that passion and hope. If you latch on to hope even when you feel like you've reached the end, energy circulates, and creation begins once again.

The greatest power that makes golfing to 100 possible, I think, is our passion and hope for life and for golf. If I have passion and hope, I'm grateful for each new day that's been given to me. I feel joy in the little things and a desire to extend the time I have left in life and in golf.

My heart is beating again like it did after establishing my life purpose when I was 30 years old. Having a reason for your heart to pound is such a great blessing! Every day that I live, I want to help at least one more person and contribute to making a better world. I want to be useful to the world anytime, anywhere. My body will age, but since I've decided to keep my mind spry like an evergreen tree, to live a life overflowing with passion until its last moment, my heart and brain feel younger than my actual age. "Keep this up, and you may really live 120 years!" I joke with myself, cheering myself on.

Golf has been with me for the first nine holes of my life. The game has let me see myself more clearly, meet good people, and get closer to nature. What other joys and pleasures will golf bring me on the back nine holes? What challenges will it present, and how will I accept and overcome them? Just imagining this fills my heart with excitement. Even when I've reached the age of 100, I hope I'll still feel a thrill of expectation the night before heading to the golf course.

It wasn't our choice to come into this world, but we can choose how to live in it. Just as we received life, we also received space and time. How I use my space and time before I leave the world is up to me. Whatever environment you're in, obstacles aren't a problem if you remember that you have a brain with bright consciousness and the power to choose. Those who live with this kind of thinking can make their birth blessed, their life art, and their death an honor.

When I was a beginner in golf, I didn't understand what people meant when they said, "The finishing posture is important." You've already hit the ball, sent it on its trajectory, so why does it matter what posture you adopt at the finish? Is it to look cool? What's more, if you haven't made a good shot, trying to adopt a fine finishing posture would be incredibly embarrassing. Only much later did I understand that a good follow-through influences the swing that comes before it and simultaneously acts as a mirror allowing me to observe the swing I've just completed.

Impact is difficult to control since it occurs in the split second when the clubhead and ball meet. Intentionally trying to control it can easily make for a bad shot. But if you accurately plan and practice your swing path from solid address to final finish, you can achieve the best impact while following that path.

The same goes for life. Who do I want to be in this life? It's not easy to make the best choices at every moment, analyzing every situation around you. An important guideline is asking yourself, "Are the choices I'm making now leading me to the finish I want, to the person I want to be when my life is done?" Remembering your finish at critical moments of choice helps you make better choices and live a more fulfilling life. Look at someone's finish in golf, and you can know their swing and ball flight. In the same way, who I am at the end of my life, and the feeling I have in my heart at that moment, tells me most clearly the sort of life I've lived.

I hope to speak these words to warm my heart when I hole out after finishing the round of my life: "Well played."

The Tao of Golf

Living for the Completion of the Soul

The most important discovery in my life was that I have a True Self. It was also realizing that everyone has such a self, not just me. We all have a True Self that can say, "My body is not me, but mine. My mind is not me, but mine." Meeting the True Self, the master of body and mind—what we can also call the soul—is the event of a lifetime.

When you meet the True Self, you can live a life of genuine independence, autonomy, and freedom. You can design and create your life independently without being led about by the environment or conditions around you. People who have encountered their genuine self are their own source of hope. They develop inner strength and passion and can also provide hope to others. Each one of us can serve as hope for the world by living as our genuine self.

You'll always feel inadequate if you only live according to the values and assessments of others. But when you feel your absolute value within through an encounter with your True Self, that value cannot be compared with anything, and you'll finally know true peace and freedom. When we live our lives realizing our absolute value, we finally feel whole. This is a life for the completion of the soul.

Completing Your Life and Welcoming Death

There's nothing in life we can own. I don't even own my own life. The life that came from nature stays with me a while before leaving me and returning to nature with my death. That's why we should confidently burn up the energy of our lives instead of trying to hang on to it. Our lives are burning every day anyway, like candle wicks. We might as well use them for some good purpose before we go on our way.

When I visited Nepal about 20 years ago, I saw something fascinating in a street shop selling Tibetan souvenirs. It was an actual human skull covered in silver foil and decorated with beads of various colors and shapes. When I asked its purpose, I learned that it was used as a container for food. I asked why anyone would eat food out of a skull and was told that it reminds us to cherish every moment and keeps us from forgetting that death is always there alongside life. Deeply moved by the Tibetan philosophy concerning death, I bought that skull bowl. It's still in my house in Sedona.

I've decided to live 120 years, playing golf my whole life, so I'm working to develop a good lifestyle and keep my body and brain in top condition. At the same time, I'm aware that death can come for me at any time. That's why I intend to cherish every day, realizing my values and living life with no regrets.

At the moment of death, I want to breathe my last breath in peace, exhaling comfortably. I want to close the final moments of my life by emptying myself, breathing out in gratitude, not by sucking in the air, ending life remorseful and afraid. I believe that living true to my soul—listening to the voice of my True Self—will make my last breath a peaceful exhalation.

Korean Sundo has the expression *Chunhwa*, meaning "becoming heaven." This refers to the death of someone who has discovered, realized, and completed his True Self. It's the peaceful, dignified death of one who knows that he's not trapped in the time between birth and death, that he has come from nature and will return to nature.

We can just exist, or we can truly live. When you awaken to and realize your true value, you cherish every moment of your life and feel alive with every cell in your body. Chunhwa is a death that can be met with calmness and gratitude at the end of such a life.

Using Our Spiritual Sense to Manage the Earth Together

Living life to discover the True Self and complete the soul is necessary not only for individuals, but also for humankind and the earth as a whole. There is hope for our planet only if humans recover their spiritual sense for cherishing and caring for life and nature.

Everyone has a spiritual sense, but it becomes obscured by emotions and desires. Feelings and desires will constantly come and go as long as you have a body. The important thing is to maintain the spiritual sense needed to manage those feelings. The True Self, the soul, is the master capable of controlling emotions and desires. Find your True Self, and you'll become aware of an observer consciousness that can detachedly watch your body and mind. Unless you sense this part of the mind that transcends your emotions—that is the master of them—you'll end up worshipping your feelings like gods. Day after day, the events and phenomena of life trigger countless emotions and reactions inside of us. Life's most important study is to find the mind that can master these feelings instead of being dragged around by them.

I think that using one's spiritual sense to manage life and take care of the earth should be common sense for people living in the 21st century. Our spiritual sense makes us feel that we're one with all life instead of exclusively belonging to a particular country, group, religion, or culture. Taking us beyond individual and collective selfishness, this spiritual sense leads us to have earth citizenship consciousness, where we naturally concern ourselves with the health and happiness of the whole planet.

If more people made our collective well-being their mission, we could make the earth a more peaceful, sustainable home. I dream of a planet where everyone is happy—and I firmly believe that humanity has the spiritual sense and power to create such a world. The goal of the rest of my life is to do everything I can to leave future generations a planet that's closer to that dream, even if only by a little.

The 100-Year Golfer

I believe that finding, developing, and expressing the value of the True Self inside each of us contributes to the health and happiness of other people and the world. This is the good life as I know it, and on the golf course, my task is to make this value, this Tao, come to life in each and every moment.

To Friends Searching for the Tao in Golf

If the essence of Tao is awakening to the relationship between the True Self and the mind, then the essence of golf is finding your own perfect swing. If you express the goals of Tao and golf as a simple diagram, you get the same picture: a round circle.

When you watch your own mind, you'll notice the rough edges designed to protect your pure heart from the world. To express your heart freely, begin rounding off the rough edges and corners of your heart so that you get caught on nothing. Golfers hone their swings just as we polish our hearts—smoothing the rough edges, allowing them to flow freely no matter what challenges they face. They repeat the process again and again until power, balance, and rhythm have come together in a swing that is entirely, genuinely their own.

The most important thing in golf is discovering your natural swing and using it in reality. Playing lifelong golf means creating a swing that matches your constitution and temperament, regardless of your age. For those who study the mind, the process of discovering and perfecting your golf swing is surprisingly similar to the process of discovering and realizing your True Self. I regularly play golf alone because I feel the Tao in this game. I want to play golf my own way, following my heart, just as I've lived my life through the Tao. I want to be able to say at any moment, "I am authentically, unapologetically me." My efforts to find and realize my unique swing will continue until the last day that I pick up a golf club.

If your purpose in golf is to find your swing, not just to score well, you'll be able to maintain your composure without being put off by desires or emotions. If you have the attitude that you'll play golf your whole life, continuing to perfect your swing rather than trying to beat someone in competition, your golf experience will be more meaningful and fulfilling. Golf's final gifts to us are not top scores but calm composure, gratitude, fond memories of the people we were with, and the satisfaction of having done our best.

Regardless of country, faith, age, sex, occupation, or social status, we become golfers the moment we pick up our golf clubs and stand on the teeing ground. The rules and courses for the game of golf were designed by people, but the ultimate partner in golf is nature, not another person. Golf is about getting to know our own bodies and minds, which are aspects of nature, and we golf within natural law, which is fair to everyone. Natural law ultimately rules the game of golf, even as we explore the potential of new technology, better swing analysis, and continued application of sports psychology.

Golf is a nature-friendly sport played in the sun, wind, air, and sometimes rain and snow. Few sports allow you to enjoy the benefits of nature as much as golf does. It's true that creating and maintaining a golf course takes a lot of resources and places a burden on the planet. As much as I love golf, I'm incurring a debt to the earth and feel a responsibility to repay it. Each time I hit the ball, I remind myself of the endless respect and gratitude we should have for our planet, which is very similar to my golf ball traveling through the expanse of space.

You may have noticed that, recently, developers in many places have been building golf courses that utilize the natural features of the land rather than artificial constructions, preserving nature as much as possible. A growing number of courses are also managing the grass without using chemical fertilizers and conserving water in order to be more ecologically responsible. I'm glad and thankful for this, and I hope the golfing world continues to develop this type of nature-friendly management.

Those who play golf together are friends who can be thought of as fellow seekers on the path of enlightenment. I hope that together we can learn the Way of Golf, the Way of Life, which is a study not only of the game we play, but of ourselves, the players. Given that there are 100 million golfers worldwide and six million in my home country of South Korea alone, the positive influence that golfers can have on society is tremendous. I hope that each time we step on a golf course, our conduct exudes the fragrance of the Tao. I hope that everyone we encounter is inspired to better manage the planet and society for the benefit of all life. May my fellow seekers enjoy a lifetime of the kind of golf that brings happiness, excitement, and the spiritual joy of encountering and realizing our True Selves.

Acknowledgments

I'm very grateful to all the people who have helped me turn my passion for golf and for assisting people to live long, fulfilling lives into a published work. It has been a happy journey, and these people were my motor.

Daniel Graham translated the Korean into English, and editors Nicole Dean and Phyllis Elving turned the translation into a text that English speakers would enjoy reading. David Driscoll did a significant amount of editing, adding his knowledge and passion for the game of golf. The talented Eunjung Shin made the illustrations for the exercises while Yeosun Park took the photographs shown throughout the book. Kiryl Lysenka and Junghee Lee gave the book character and structure with their cover and interior design. And I always appreciate the staff at my American publisher, Best Life Media.

I'm also grateful to the several golfers in South Korea and the United States who shared their own stories of applying Brain Education to their golf game. And I appreciate all the people who gave their honest opinion on the manuscript during several stages of the process.

About the Author

Ilchi Lee is a visionary, mentor, and educator who has devoted his life to teaching energy principles and developing methods to nurture the full potential of the human brain.

For the last four decades, his mission has been to help people harness their creative power. For this goal, he developed mind-body training methods such as Body & Brain Yoga and Brain Education, which have inspired many people worldwide to live healthier and happier lives. He also founded the undergraduate Global Cyber University and the graduate University of Brain Education.

Lee has penned more than 40 books, including the *New York Times* bestseller *The Call of Sedona: Journey of the Heart*, and *I've Decided to Live 120 Years: The Ancient Secret to Longevity, Vitality, and Life Transformation*.

A well-respected humanitarian, Ilchi Lee has worked with the United Nations and other organizations for global peace through his nonprofit International Brain Education Association (IBREA Foundation). In addition, he began the Earth Citizen Movement, a global drive to raise awareness of living mindfully and sustainably as a steward of the earth, and started the nonprofit Earth Citizens Organization (ECO). For more information about Ilchi Lee, visit Ilchi.com.

Resources

Ilchi Brain Golf YouTube Channel

This channel brings the advice in *The 100-Year Golfer* into a video format. Find how-to's, personal stories, and other golf tips given by a long-time Brain Education instructor and passionate golfer David Driscoll. Watch and subscribe at YouTube.com/IlchiBrainGolf.

Body & Brain Yoga and Tai Chi Classes

Find classes with expert instructors in the exercises in this book at Body & Brain Yoga Tai Chi centers. There are approximately 100 Body & Brain Yoga Tai Chi centers across the United States, with more centers in South Korea, Japan, Europe, Canada, and New Zealand. Group classes, workshops, and individual sessions are available both online and offline. Find a U.S. center near you at BodynBrain.com.

Ilchi Lee's Email Newsletter

Ilchi Lee sends weekly inspirational messages, tips, and meditations to manage your body and mind to master your life. Get ongoing advice for connecting with your natural rhythm and how to apply Brain Education to your life. Sign up at Ilchi.com/newsletter.

Books of Related Interest

The following books can also help you enjoy golf and good health for the rest of your life. See them all and more of Ilchi Lee's books at BestLifeMedia.com.

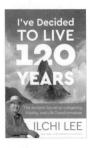

I've Decided to Live 120 Years
The Ancient Secret to Longevity, Vitality, and Life Transformation

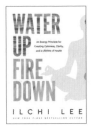

Water Up Fire Down
An Energy Principle for Creating Calmness, Clarity, and a Lifetime of Health

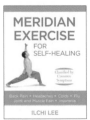

Meridian Exercise for Self Healing
Classified by Common Symptoms

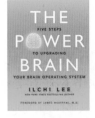

The Power Brain
Five Steps to Upgrading Your Brain Operating System

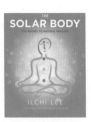

The Solar Body
The Secret to Natural Healing

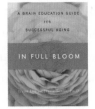

In Full Bloom
A Brain Education Guide for Successful Aging

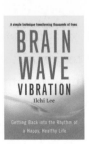

Brain Wave Vibration
Getting Back into the Rhythm of a Happy, Healthy Life

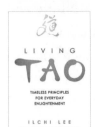

Living Tao
Timeless Principles for Everyday Enlightenment

The 100-Year Golfer

Ilchi Brain Golf
YouTube Channel